# UNDERSTANDING ARTHRITIS

## A Guide to Managing and Living with Joint Pain and Inflammation

### Kian M. Hart

# Table of Contents

First Printed 2023.

ISBN:

DIGITAL VERSION: 978-1-77684-811-9

PHYSICAL VERSION: 978-1-77684-702-0

• A New Zealand Designed Product

**Get A Free Book At: go.xspurts.com/free-book-offer[4]**

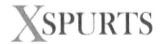

5

---

1. https://Xspurts.com

2. https://Xspurts.com

3. https://Xspurts.com

**4. https://go.xspurts.com/free-book-offer**

5. https://xspurts.com/

# Introduction

Welcome, fellow adventurers, to the fascinating realm of Understanding Arthritis! Join me on this informative and lighthearted expedition as we delve into the intricacies of this condition and discover ways to conquer its challenges. Prepare yourself for a journey filled with knowledge, a dash of humor, and a quest for relief!

Arthritis, affectionately known as the "joint party crasher," is a condition that can turn even the most graceful dancers into wobbly penguins. It's like a mischievous trickster that sneaks into our joints and throws a wild party, leaving us with pain, stiffness, and sometimes a few questionable dance moves.

But fear not, fellow adventurers, for we are armed with knowledge to navigate this bumpy joint journey. So, let's strap on our joint-supporting armor and embark on this adventure together!

Arthritis, which is derived from the Greek words "arthro" meaning joint and "itis" meaning inflammation, is not a single condition but a vast galaxy of conditions affecting the joints. From the mighty warriors like osteoarthritis and rheumatoid arthritis to the lesser-known cosmic entities like psoriatic arthritis and gout, each form of arthritis has its own quirks and battle strategies.

Now, let's dive deeper into the causes of this joint rebellion. Aging, like a cosmic clock ticking away, is a prominent factor in the development of arthritis. But don't fret, for arthritis can also strike younger adventurers, much like a surprise meteor shower. Other cosmic culprits may include genetics, joint injuries, and cosmic immune system malfunctions.

As we explore the vast cosmos of arthritis, it's essential to understand its various signs and symptoms. Picture this: your joints becoming as creaky as a cosmic pirate ship, mornings feeling as slow as cosmic molasses, and the occasional joint swelling that makes you wonder if you've stumbled into a cosmic balloon festival. These are just a few of the cosmic clues that may indicate the presence of arthritis.

Now, let's add a sprinkle of humor to our cosmic journey. Imagine your joints as mischievous cosmic tricksters, playing hide-and-seek with your keys or making you drop things at the most inconvenient times. But fear not, for a little humor can be the cosmic glue that holds us together on this adventure.

But what can we do to combat these cosmic joint invaders? Fear not, for there are cosmic remedies and strategies available to help manage arthritis symptoms and reclaim your cosmic mobility. From gentle exercises and stretches to cosmic hot and cold treatments, there's a cosmic arsenal of tools to alleviate discomfort and keep those joints cosmic.

Additionally, exploring the cosmic realm of medications, under the guidance of a cosmic healthcare provider, can offer relief from pain and inflammation. Nonsteroidal anti-inflammatory drugs (NSAIDs), disease-modifying antirheumatic drugs (DMARDs), and cosmic corticosteroids are just a few cosmic potions in the battle against arthritis.

But let's not forget the cosmic power of self-care. Proper nutrition, stress management, and cosmic rest can be our allies in this joint venture. Think of it as pampering your joints with cosmic spa treatments and ensuring they stay in tip-top shape for your cosmic adventures.

As we embark on this cosmic journey through Understanding Arthritis, remember that knowledge and a cosmic sense of humor will be our guides. Together, let's explore the cosmos of arthritis, seek relief, and conquer the challenges that come our way. Safe travels, fellow adventurers, and may your joints dance with cosmic grace once more!

# What is arthritis?

Welcome to the enlightening world of Understanding Arthritis, where joints take on a life of their own and embark on unexpected adventures. Arthritis, derived from the Greek words "arthro" (meaning joint) and "itis" (meaning inflammation), is a mischievous condition that loves to throw a party in our joints. It's like having a group of rowdy gatecrashers wreaking havoc and leaving behind pain, stiffness, and some interesting dance moves.

Now, let's delve into the cosmic nature of arthritis. Picture your joints as a bustling city, complete with roads, buildings, and inhabitants. But when arthritis strikes, it's as if a construction crew has suddenly invaded, causing chaos and inflammation within the joint infrastructure.

There are numerous types of arthritis, each with its own cosmic flair. Osteoarthritis, the most common form, is like the wise elder of the cosmic joint community. It's often associated with wear and tear, as if the joints have been on a never-ending roller coaster ride. Rheumatoid arthritis, on the other hand, is a bit more rebellious, as if the immune system has declared war on the joints, launching cosmic missiles of inflammation.

Psoriatic arthritis adds a touch of cosmic intrigue, joining forces with the skin condition psoriasis to create a cosmic tag team of joint and skin mischief. And let's not forget the cosmic gout, which feels like tiny crystals have invaded the joints, causing sudden, intense pain akin to being stung by cosmic bees.

But fear not, for in this cosmic battle against arthritis, there are allies we can call upon. Physical therapy, the cosmic equivalent of joint boot camp, can help improve joint mobility and strengthen the cosmic support structures. Think of it as sending your joints to a cosmic fitness retreat.

Medications also play a crucial role in our cosmic fight against arthritis. Nonsteroidal anti-inflammatory drugs (NSAIDs) act like cosmic pacifiers, soothing the joint inflammation. Disease-modifying antirheumatic drugs (DMARDs) are the cosmic superheroes that target the immune system, fighting off the cosmic inflammation. And for those moments when pain reaches cosmic levels, corticosteroids swoop in like cosmic pain relievers.

Let's not forget the cosmic powers of heat and cold. Heat therapy, like a warm cosmic embrace, can help soothe joint stiffness and relax the cosmic tension. Cold therapy, on the other hand, acts as a cosmic chill pill, reducing inflammation and numbing the cosmic pain.

But perhaps the most cosmic weapon of all is knowledge. Understanding your specific type of arthritis and its cosmic tendencies can empower you to make informed decisions and take control of your cosmic joints. Educate yourself about the cosmic triggers that worsen your symptoms and the cosmic strategies that provide relief.

In conclusion, arthritis is a cosmic adventure that takes place within the realm of our joints. It can come in various cosmic forms, each with its own unique traits and quirks. However, with the right cosmic allies, such as physical therapy and medications, and a cosmic understanding of our condition, we can navigate this cosmic journey with grace and humor. Remember, when arthritis tries to throw a cosmic party in your joints, it's up to you to show it who's boss and bring the cosmic dance moves back to the floor.

# Overview of symptoms and diagnosis

Welcome to the enlightening cosmic journey of Understanding Arthritis, where our joints sometimes act like divas with a flair for drama. Arthritis is a condition that can turn even the most graceful joint movements into a cosmic performance worthy of an audience.

When it comes to symptoms, arthritis has its own unique cosmic language. The first cosmic cue is pain, which can range from a gentle cosmic whisper to a full-blown cosmic opera. Joints may feel achy, tender, or as if they're being put through a cosmic workout they didn't sign up for.

Stiffness is another cosmic side effect of arthritis. Imagine your joints as cosmic door hinges that haven't been oiled in eons. They may resist movement, making you feel like a cosmic statue in need of a little cosmic WD-4

Swelling can also crash the cosmic party. Picture your joints as balloons filled with cosmic fluid. When arthritis joins the festivities, these cosmic balloons can inflate, causing joint swelling that would make any circus proud.

But how do we diagnose this cosmic condition? Well, doctors have a cosmic bag of tricks to unravel the mystery. They may start with a thorough examination of your joints, like cosmic detectives searching for clues. X-rays can capture cosmic images of your joints, revealing any cosmic mischief happening beneath the surface.

Blood tests are like cosmic interrogations, seeking answers from the cosmic suspects. They can detect specific markers that indicate the presence of arthritis, ruling out other cosmic imposters.

In some cases, doctors may even suggest a cosmic journey into your joint space through a procedure called arthroscopy. It's like sending a tiny cosmic spaceship equipped with a camera to explore the cosmic wonders within your joints.

Now, let's not forget the different cosmic characters of arthritis. Osteoarthritis, the most common form, often plays the role of the wise cosmic elder. It's like the joint version of a vintage cosmic record, with wear and tear being its cosmic groove.

Rheumatoid arthritis, on the other hand, is the cosmic rebel with an immune system that goes rogue. It's like having a cosmic rock band playing an eternal concert in your joints, complete with pyrotechnics of inflammation.

There are other cosmic actors in this cosmic theater as well. Gout, with its crystal-like deposits, can feel like stepping on cosmic Legos. Psoriatic arthritis, a cosmic collaboration with the skin condition psoriasis, adds an artistic touch of cosmic mischief to the joint performance.

In conclusion, understanding the cosmic symptoms and diagnosis of arthritis is like deciphering a cosmic code. Pain, stiffness, and swelling are the cosmic signals that something may be amiss in the joint universe. With the help of cosmic examinations, imaging, and blood tests, doctors can identify the cosmic culprit behind your joint troubles.

So, embrace your cosmic role as a detective in the cosmic mystery of arthritis. Remember, the cosmic characters of arthritis each have their own unique quirks. Together, we can uncover the cosmic secrets of this condition and embark on a cosmic journey towards relief and better joint health.

# The impact of arthritis on daily life

Welcome to the cosmic carnival of Understanding Arthritis, where joints sometimes throw unexpected twists and turns into the cosmic dance of daily life. Arthritis, with its unique flair for surprises, can bring about a cosmic symphony of challenges that make even the simplest tasks feel like a celestial odyssey.

The impact of arthritis on daily life can be likened to a cosmic roller coaster ride. Imagine waking up in the morning, ready to tackle the cosmic challenges ahead, only to be greeted by stiff joints that feel as if they've been exploring the outer reaches of the universe overnight. Suddenly, putting on socks becomes a cosmic balancing act worthy of a tightrope walker.

Simple activities like opening jars can transform into cosmic battles, where gripping becomes a test of cosmic strength and determination. You might find yourself resorting to ingenious cosmic techniques like using rubber gloves or cosmic tools to conquer the stubborn lids.

Arthritis has a way of adding cosmic spice to even the most mundane tasks. Picture this: you're enjoying a cosmic dinner with friends, and the cosmic meal is served. But as you reach for the celestial cutlery, a cosmic pain shoots through your hand, turning the act of dining into a cosmic culinary challenge. It's like trying to eat a cosmic feast with an alien hand.

Mobility can also be affected by the cosmic whims of arthritis. The cosmic dance of walking may become an unpredictable performance, where joints creak and protest with each step. You might find yourself mastering the art of cosmic improvisation, adjusting your stride or seeking cosmic props like canes or walkers to navigate the cosmic terrain.

Sleep, that sacred cosmic ritual, may also be disrupted by arthritis. As you settle into your cosmic sanctuary, joint pain can transform your cosmic bed into a battleground. It's like trying to find comfort on a cosmic asteroid field. But fear not, there are cosmic pillows and mattresses designed to cradle your joints and bring about a peaceful cosmic slumber.

Social interactions can also be impacted by arthritis. Imagine attending a cosmic gathering, filled with laughter and cosmic merriment. But as you join in the festivities, the cosmic pain intensifies, and you find yourself searching for cosmic excuses to retreat from the cosmic revelry. It's like being a cosmic party pooper against your own will.

However, amidst the cosmic challenges, there is always room for humor. Arthritis teaches us to find laughter in the face of cosmic adversity. We become cosmic comedians, sharing stories of cosmic mishaps and creative solutions to everyday cosmic challenges. Laughter becomes our cosmic superpower, providing a sense of cosmic resilience and reminding us not to take life's cosmic hurdles too seriously.

In conclusion, the impact of arthritis on daily life can be both cosmic and comical. It presents us with unexpected twists and turns, transforming routine activities into cosmic adventures. But with cosmic creativity, a dash of humor, and cosmic adaptations, we can navigate this cosmic journey with grace and resilience. So, let's embrace the cosmic challenges, find cosmic humor in the cosmic mishaps, and create our own cosmic narrative of living well with arthritis.

# Understanding Arthritis Types

Welcome to the vibrant world of Understanding Arthritis Types, where joints come in all shapes, sizes, and cosmic personalities. Arthritis, like a cosmic kaleidoscope, presents us with a dazzling array of types, each with its unique characteristics and quirks. So, fasten your seatbelts as we embark on a cosmic journey to explore the cosmic cast of arthritis characters.

First up on our cosmic tour is the dazzling rheumatoid arthritis, the cosmic diva of the joint world. With its cosmic flair for drama, it loves to surprise its hosts with symmetrical joint pain and inflammation. It's like a cosmic symphony of joint rebellion, where both sides of the body join in unison to perform a cosmic protest. But fear not, with the right cosmic treatment and cosmic interventions, this celestial diva can be tamed.

Next, we encounter the mighty osteoarthritis, the cosmic elder of the joint family. This wise cosmic sage slowly wears down the protective cosmic cartilage, causing joints to become stiff and achy. It's like witnessing the cosmic erosion of a celestial masterpiece. But fret not, with cosmic care and cosmic lifestyle modifications, we can find cosmic harmony in the face of this cosmic sage.

Enter the cosmic gout, the mischievous trickster of the joint universe. It delights in surprising its hosts with sudden and intense joint pain, often targeting the cosmic big toe. It's like a cosmic game of hide-and-seek, where the gouty joint hides in plain sight, waiting to spring its cosmic surprise. But fear not, with cosmic medication and cosmic dietary changes, this celestial trickster can be kept at bay.

Now, let's meet the cosmic ankylosing spondylitis, the cosmic backbone of the arthritis world. This cosmic character loves to make its presence known in the spine, causing stiffness and fusion of the cosmic vertebrae. It's like witnessing a celestial dance of the spine, where flexibility gives way to cosmic rigidity. But worry not, with cosmic exercise and cosmic medications, we can keep the cosmic backbone strong and supple.

Last but not least, we encounter the cosmic psoriatic arthritis, the cosmic artist of the joint realm. With its cosmic connection to psoriasis, it paints a cosmic masterpiece of joint inflammation and skin flare-ups. It's like witnessing a cosmic collaboration of art and science, where the canvas becomes the joint. But fret not, with cosmic medications and cosmic skin care, we can bring balance to this cosmic collaboration.

As we conclude our cosmic tour of arthritis types, we realize that each cosmic character brings its own set of challenges and cosmic opportunities. But in this cosmic tapestry of arthritis, we find unity in our shared journey of cosmic resilience. Together, we can navigate the cosmic twists and turns, armed with cosmic treatments, cosmic adaptations, and a sprinkle of cosmic humor.

So, whether you're in the cosmic realm of rheumatoid arthritis, the cosmic domain of osteoarthritis, or any other cosmic corner of the joint universe, remember that you're not alone. With cosmic healthcare providers, cosmic support systems, and a dash of cosmic humor, we can embrace the cosmic variety of arthritis types and live our lives to the fullest.

In the cosmic dance of arthritis, let us celebrate our cosmic diversity, find strength in our cosmic similarities, and create a cosmic narrative of understanding and compassion. Together, we can paint a cosmic masterpiece of resilience, where arthritis becomes just another colorful thread in the cosmic fabric of our lives.

# Osteoarthritis

Welcome to the world of Osteoarthritis, where joints take on a journey of wear and tear, and a sprinkle of cosmic humor. Osteoarthritis, often referred to as the "wear and tear" arthritis, is like the wise elder of the joint family, reminding us that with age comes wisdom and a few creaks and cracks.

Imagine your joints as cosmic machinery, tirelessly working day in and day out to keep you moving. But over time, the cosmic gears and cosmic cartilage that cushion your joints begin to show signs of cosmic wear and tear. It's like a celestial symphony of squeaks and groans, reminding you of the cosmic journey your joints have taken.

Osteoarthritis, the cosmic sage, primarily affects the weight-bearing joints such as the knees, hips, and spine. It's like witnessing a cosmic dance of balance and gravity, where the weight of the world takes its toll on the cosmic joints. But fear not, with a little cosmic care and cosmic lifestyle adjustments, we can find harmony in the cosmic dance.

As the cosmic cartilage starts to break down, joints become stiff, achy, and sometimes swollen. It's like experiencing a cosmic rust in the cosmic machinery, where movement becomes a little more challenging. But worry not, with cosmic exercises and cosmic physical therapy, we can keep the cosmic joints well-oiled and the cosmic rust at bay.

One of the cosmic quirks of osteoarthritis is its affinity for chilly weather. It's like the cosmic joints have their own weather forecast, predicting cosmic discomfort when the temperature drops. So, when the cosmic winter comes knocking, be prepared with a cosmic blanket of warmth and a dash of cosmic humor to weather the storm.

In the cosmic realm of osteoarthritis, weight management takes center stage. Maintaining a healthy weight is like lightening the cosmic load on your joints, giving them a cosmic breather and a chance to thrive. So, grab your cosmic sneakers, embark on cosmic walks, and let the cosmic pounds melt away.

But let's not forget the cosmic power of medication. From cosmic pain relievers to cosmic anti-inflammatory drugs, they offer a cosmic respite from discomfort and help us keep the cosmic spring in our steps. Just remember to consult your cosmic healthcare provider to find the right cosmic prescription for you.

As we journey through the cosmic landscape of osteoarthritis, let's embrace the cosmic adaptations. From cosmic assistive devices like canes and braces to cosmic ergonomic modifications in our daily lives, we can create a cosmic environment that supports our joints and allows us to navigate the cosmic challenges with grace and a pinch of cosmic humor.

In the cosmic tapestry of arthritis, osteoarthritis is like the cosmic reminder to cherish our joints and give them the cosmic care they deserve. So, whether it's cosmic hot packs, cosmic gentle stretches, or cosmic massages, let's pamper our joints and remind them of the cosmic appreciation they deserve.

As we conclude our cosmic exploration of osteoarthritis, let us remember that it's not just about the cosmic joints but also the cosmic mindset. Embrace the cosmic wisdom of the cosmic sage, find humor in the cosmic creaks, and live your life to the fullest, one cosmic step at a time.

# Rheumatoid arthritis

Welcome to the world of Rheumatoid Arthritis, where joints embark on a cosmic battle against their own cosmic immune system. Rheumatoid Arthritis, or RA for short, is like the mischievous trickster in the realm of arthritis, playing cosmic pranks on the unsuspecting joints.

In this cosmic game, the body's immune system gets a little confused and starts attacking the cosmic joints as if they were cosmic invaders. It's like the immune system has its own cosmic version of hide-and-seek, mistakenly identifying the joints as the hidden cosmic enemies.

RA loves to surprise its victims with morning stiffness and joint pain, as if playing a cosmic game of "Guess Who?" where the joints are the unwilling players. But fear not, with cosmic medications and cosmic treatments, we can minimize the cosmic mischief and restore harmony to the cosmic joints.

The cosmic joints affected by RA can be quite capricious, showing up in a symphony of swelling, redness, and warmth. It's like the cosmic joints are having their own disco party, with pulsating beats of inflammation. But worry not, with the help of cosmic anti-inflammatory medications, we can turn down the cosmic music and bring tranquility back to the joints.

One of the quirks of RA is its cosmic preference for symmetry. It's like the cosmic joints have their own cosmic twin, experiencing similar cosmic discomfort on both sides of the body. So, when the cosmic left knee throws a tantrum, the cosmic right knee decides to join the party too.

RA is like the cosmic master of disguise, sometimes hiding behind the mask of fatigue and general malaise. It's like the cosmic villain wearing a cloak, trying to exhaust its victims with cosmic weariness. But let's not be fooled, with proper cosmic self-care, rest, and a dash of cosmic humor, we can conquer the cosmic fatigue.

In the cosmic battle against RA, medications play a crucial role. From cosmic disease-modifying antirheumatic drugs (DMARDs) to cosmic biologic agents, they act as the cosmic superheroes, fighting against the cosmic inflammation and protecting the joints. But remember, consult your cosmic healthcare provider to find the right cosmic treatment plan for you.

Living with RA requires cosmic adaptation. From cosmic joint protection techniques to cosmic assistive devices, we can create a cosmic environment that supports our joints and eases the cosmic burden. So, embrace the cosmic splendor of wrist splints, knee braces, and ergonomic tools, and let them be your cosmic allies in this battle.

As we navigate the cosmic realm of RA, let's not forget the importance of cosmic self-care. A cosmic diet rich in anti-inflammatory foods, regular cosmic exercise, and stress management can be our cosmic weapons against the cosmic inflammation. So, enjoy a cosmic dance class, savor cosmic blueberries, and find cosmic Zen in a moment of relaxation.

In the cosmic tapestry of arthritis, Rheumatoid Arthritis is the cosmic trickster, reminding us to stay vigilant and adapt to its cosmic pranks. But with the right cosmic strategies, a touch of cosmic humor, and the support of your cosmic healthcare team, you can lead a fulfilling life and triumph over the cosmic mischief of RA.

# Psoriatic arthritis

Welcome to the world of Psoriatic Arthritis, where joints and skin join forces to create a cosmic collaboration that keeps us on our toes. Psoriatic Arthritis, or PsA for short, is like the cosmic duo of arthritis and psoriasis, teaming up to make their presence known.

Picture this: joints and skin are like cosmic roommates, sharing the same space and occasionally getting into cosmic quarrels. It's like a cosmic sitcom, where the joints and skin take turns playing pranks on each other.

PsA has a flair for the dramatic, showcasing its cosmic abilities by causing joint pain, swelling, and stiffness. It's like the cosmic performer stealing the spotlight and demanding attention. But fear not, with the help of cosmic medications and cosmic treatments, we can bring harmony back to the cosmic stage.

The cosmic skin in PsA plays its own role in this cosmic drama. It's like a cosmic canvas, with patches of red, scaly skin appearing out of nowhere. It's as if the skin has its own cosmic graffiti artist, creating unique and unpredictable patterns. But worry not, cosmic topical treatments and cosmic medications can calm the cosmic chaos and restore the cosmic canvas.

PsA is like the cosmic chameleon, changing its appearance and symptoms over time. It can be a cosmic trickster, affecting different joints or different areas of the skin. It's like playing cosmic hide-and-seek, where PsA keeps us guessing. But with the cosmic guidance of healthcare providers, we can adapt and navigate the cosmic twists and turns.

One of the unique aspects of PsA is its cosmic affinity for the nails. It's like the cosmic manicurist has a mischievous side, leaving behind pitted and discolored nails as their cosmic signature. But don't worry, cosmic nail care and cosmic treatments can help us maintain cosmic beauty.

Living with PsA requires cosmic teamwork. From cosmic rheumatologists to cosmic dermatologists, healthcare providers work together to develop a cosmic treatment plan that addresses both the joint and skin aspects of PsA. So, embrace the cosmic collaboration and let your healthcare team be your cosmic partners in this journey.

PsA also reminds us of the importance of cosmic self-care. A cosmic balanced diet, regular cosmic exercise, and stress management can be our cosmic allies in managing the cosmic symptoms. So, indulge in cosmic healthy foods, embark on cosmic yoga adventures, and find cosmic tranquility in moments of relaxation.

In the cosmic realm of PsA, medication can play a vital role. Cosmic disease-modifying antirheumatic drugs (DMARDs), cosmic biologic agents, and cosmic targeted therapies are like the cosmic superheroes, fighting against the cosmic inflammation and protecting our cosmic joints and skin. But remember, consult your cosmic healthcare provider to find the right cosmic treatment plan for you.

As we navigate the cosmic collaboration of PsA, let's not forget the importance of cosmic support. Connect with cosmic support groups, seek cosmic guidance from healthcare professionals, and lean on your cosmic loved ones for cosmic understanding and encouragement.

In the cosmic tapestry of arthritis, Psoriatic Arthritis is the cosmic duo, reminding us to appreciate the cosmic connection between joints and skin. With the right cosmic strategies, a touch of cosmic humor, and the support of your cosmic team, you can lead a fulfilling life and find beauty even in the cosmic collaboration of PsA.

# Gout

Welcome to the wild world of Gout, where joints and crystals engage in a celestial dance that can make you feel like you're walking on stardust. Gout is like the cosmic rebel of arthritis, causing sudden and intense bouts of pain that can catch you off guard.

Imagine your joints as cosmic nightclubs, where urate crystals like to party and cause trouble. They're like unruly cosmic guests who overstay their welcome, causing chaos and inflammation. But fear not, with the right cosmic strategies, we can kick these cosmic troublemakers out of the club.

Gout has a knack for striking when you least expect it, often targeting the big toe joint like a cosmic sniper. It's like a cosmic prankster, reminding you to always expect the unexpected. But fret not, with cosmic medications and cosmic lifestyle changes, we can keep these cosmic surprises at bay.

One of the cosmic culprits behind gout is none other than our cosmic diet. Foods high in purines, like red meat and seafood, are like the cosmic chefs creating the perfect recipe for a gout flare-up. It's as if they're playing a cosmic joke on us, enticing us with delicious dishes only to leave us with cosmic joint pain. But don't worry, with cosmic dietary modifications, we can still enjoy cosmic culinary delights without inviting the cosmic gout to the party.

Gout has a peculiar sense of timing, often choosing the most inconvenient moments to strike. It's like the cosmic troublemaker who crashes your cosmic vacation or shows up uninvited to a cosmic party. But fret not, cosmic planning and preparation can help us navigate these cosmic surprises and enjoy life to the fullest.

When gout strikes, it can feel like a cosmic battle. The joint becomes swollen, red, and excruciatingly painful. It's like a cosmic battlefield, with the immune system and crystals engaging in a cosmic showdown. But with cosmic anti-inflammatory medications and cosmic icing techniques, we can calm the cosmic chaos and restore peace to the joint.

The cosmic secret to managing gout lies in hydration. Drinking plenty of water is like the cosmic cleansing ritual, flushing out the cosmic urate crystals and keeping them at bay. It's like giving the cosmic troublemakers a one-way ticket out of your joints.

Gout reminds us to pay attention to our cosmic lifestyle choices. Limiting alcohol consumption, maintaining a healthy weight, and engaging in regular cosmic exercise can be our cosmic allies in preventing gout flare-ups. It's like creating a cosmic fortress, protecting our joints from the cosmic infiltrators.

Living with gout requires cosmic vigilance. Keeping track of cosmic triggers, like certain foods or medications, can help us stay one step ahead of the cosmic gout attacks. It's like playing cosmic detective, uncovering the clues that lead to a pain free life.

As we navigate the cosmic terrain of gout, let's not forget the importance of cosmic support. Seek guidance from healthcare professionals, join cosmic support groups, and lean on your cosmic loved ones for understanding and encouragement.

In the cosmic realm of arthritis, Gout is the unruly rebel, reminding us to tread carefully and make cosmic choices. With the right cosmic strategies, a touch of cosmic humor, and the support of your cosmic team, you can dance through life with grace and keep the cosmic gout at bay.

# Arthritis Causes and Risk Factors

Arthritis, the cosmic mischief-maker of the joint world, has a variety of causes and risk factors that can make even the most stoic joint quiver in fear. While it may seem like arthritis randomly selects its victims, there are certain cosmic forces at play that increase the likelihood of joint troubles.

One of the cosmic culprits behind arthritis is good old age. Time, that mischievous cosmic trickster, has a way of wearing down our joints like an overplayed vinyl record. As the years go by, the cosmic wear and tear take their toll, leaving joints vulnerable to the cosmic forces of arthritis. It's like a cosmic game of Russian roulette, where time determines the winners and losers in the joint department.

But age isn't the only cosmic conspirator. Genetics, those cosmic DNA architects, can play a significant role in determining your cosmic joint destiny. If you've inherited cosmic genes that make you prone to arthritis, it's like being dealt a less than ideal cosmic hand in the card game of life. But fear not, with cosmic awareness and proactive measures, you can still shuffle the cosmic deck in your favor.

The cosmic battlefield of inflammation is another realm where arthritis gains its power. When the immune system goes haywire, attacking cosmic invaders with cosmic fervor, it can inadvertently cause damage to the joints. It's like a cosmic case of friendly fire, where the immune system's intentions are noble, but the joint pays the cosmic price. Understanding and managing inflammation is key to keeping the cosmic arthritis forces at bay.

Lifestyle choices, those cosmic forks in the road, can also influence your joint's cosmic destiny. Cosmic villains like a sedentary lifestyle and poor cosmic dietary choices can fuel the cosmic flames of arthritis. It's like being the star of your own cosmic reality show, where your actions determine the plot twists and joint outcomes. But don't worry, with cosmic exercise and a balanced cosmic diet, you can become the hero of your joint's cosmic tale.

Injuries, those cosmic accidents waiting to happen, can also be a contributing factor to the development of arthritis. Whether it's a cosmic sports mishap or a cosmic fall down the stairs, joint trauma can leave a lasting impact on your cosmic joint health. It's like a cosmic warning sign, reminding us to be cautious and protect our joints from unnecessary cosmic harm.

Certain occupations can put you at a higher risk of cosmic joint troubles. Jobs that involve repetitive cosmic movements or joint strain, like construction work or cosmic dance choreography, can wear down the joints over time. It's like a cosmic career choice that comes with both rewards and risks. But fear not, cosmic ergonomics and proper cosmic body mechanics can help you navigate the cosmic occupational hazards.

Lastly, gender can play a role in the cosmic arthritis equation. Women, those cosmic multitaskers, are more likely to experience certain types of arthritis, like rheumatoid arthritis. It's like a cosmic badge of honor for their cosmic ability to juggle the demands of life. But don't fret, cosmic ladies, with cosmic knowledge and proactive cosmic measures, you can keep the cosmic arthritis forces in check.

In the cosmic landscape of arthritis causes and risk factors, a combination of age, genetics, inflammation, lifestyle choices, injuries, occupations, and gender can shape your cosmic joint destiny. By understanding these cosmic factors and taking cosmic action, you can tilt the cosmic odds in your favor and pave the way for a joint-friendly cosmic journey.

# Age and genetics

Age and genetics, the cosmic duo that can make or break your joints' cosmic destiny. They play a significant role in determining whether you'll be swinging on cosmic dance floors or hobbling on cosmic canes.

First, let's talk about age, that sneaky cosmic trickster that gradually reveals its hand in the game of joint health. As we journey through the cosmic dance of life, our joints experience the wear and tear of cosmic activities. It's like a cosmic marathon, and our joints are the runners trying to keep up with the pace. As the cosmic odometer ticks away, the joints face the cosmic challenge of maintaining their cosmic smoothness and flexibility. However, with the passing of cosmic time, the joints may experience a natural decline in their cosmic performance. It's like a cosmic sign that reminds us to cherish our youthful cosmic joint days and take proactive cosmic measures to support our joints as they gracefully age.

Now let's meet genetics, the cosmic architects of our joint structure. Our cosmic DNA holds the blueprint that determines the strength, stability, and resilience of our joints. It's like a cosmic recipe for joint health, handed down from generation to generation. However, just as our cosmic family tree can gift us with cosmic talents, it can also bestow upon us certain cosmic vulnerabilities. If our cosmic DNA carries the cosmic codes for arthritis, it's like receiving a cosmic challenge card in the game of joint health. But fret not, cosmic knowledge is power, and by understanding our cosmic genetic predispositions, we can take proactive cosmic measures to support our joints and keep the cosmic arthritis forces at bay.

Age and genetics often team up in the cosmic dance of joint health. As we age, our cosmic genetic predispositions may become more apparent, and the cosmic wear and tear on our joints may take a toll. It's like a cosmic partnership that can either lead to cosmic harmony or cosmic joint discord. However, don't despair, for the cosmic dance floor is not solely under their command. There are cosmic steps we can take to defy their cosmic influence.

Regular cosmic exercise can be our secret weapon in the battle against age and genetics. It's like a cosmic lubricant that keeps our joints moving smoothly and counteracts the cosmic stiffness that may come with age. By engaging in low-impact cosmic activities, such as swimming, yoga, or cosmic dance, we can keep our joints supple and strong. It's like a cosmic workout that defies the gravitational pull of cosmic joint troubles.

A cosmic diet rich in anti-inflammatory foods can also be our ally. It's like a cosmic feast that nourishes our joints from the inside out. Incorporating cosmic omega-3 fatty acids, colorful fruits and vegetables, and whole grains into our cosmic plate can provide the cosmic ammunition needed to fight off the cosmic inflammation that may arise from our genetic predispositions.

So, age and genetics may have their cosmic roles in shaping our joint health, but they are not the sole dictators of our cosmic joint destiny. With the right cosmic moves, including regular exercise, a healthy cosmic diet, and cosmic awareness, we can defy their cosmic influence and enjoy cosmic dance parties well into our golden years. Remember, age is just a cosmic number, and genetics are cosmic clues, but the power to maintain healthy joints lies within us. So let's put on our cosmic dancing shoes and show age and genetics that we're ready to boogie on the cosmic dance floor of life!

# Lifestyle factors

Lifestyle factors, the cosmic influencers of our joint health. They can either be our cosmic partners in crime or our cosmic allies in the battle against arthritis. From cosmic diet choices to cosmic exercise habits, our lifestyle decisions play a significant role in determining the cosmic fate of our joints.

Let's start with the cosmic diet. Just like choosing the right cosmic fuel for our spaceship, selecting the right cosmic foods can have a profound impact on our joint health. Consuming a well-balanced cosmic diet rich in cosmic nutrients can provide our joints with the cosmic building blocks they need to thrive. Omega-3 fatty acids found in cosmic fish like salmon and cosmic walnuts have anti-inflammatory powers that can help soothe cosmic joint inflammation. And let's not forget about the cosmic superheroes known as antioxidants, found in cosmic berries and colorful cosmic vegetables. They fight the cosmic villains called free radicals, protecting our joints from cosmic damage. So, next time you're grocery shopping, think cosmic superhero squad and load up on cosmic fruits, vegetables, and cosmic whole grains to give your joints the cosmic support they deserve.

Now, let's talk about the cosmic dance of exercise. Regular cosmic movement is like a lubricant for our joints, keeping them cosmic supple and agile. But here's the cosmic catch: finding the right balance between cosmic movement and cosmic rest is key. Too much cosmic strain on our joints can lead to cosmic wear and tear, while too little cosmic movement can lead to cosmic stiffness. The cosmic sweet spot lies in low-impact cosmic activities like swimming, cycling, or even a cosmic stroll in the park. So, let's find our cosmic rhythm and keep our joints grooving to the beat of cosmic fitness.

Cosmic stress, the silent villain that can wreak havoc on our joints. It's like a cosmic pressure cooker that turns up the heat on cosmic inflammation. But fear not, we have the cosmic power to manage it. Finding cosmic stress management techniques that work for us, whether it's cosmic meditation, cosmic yoga, or cosmic deep breathing, can help us keep our cosmic cool and protect our joints from the cosmic fire of inflammation. So, let's take a cosmic pause, breathe in the cosmic calmness, and exhale the cosmic stress.

Cosmic weight management, the cosmic balancing act of gravitational forces on our joints. Maintaining a healthy cosmic weight can alleviate the cosmic burden on our joints, reducing the risk of cosmic arthritis. It's like giving our joints a cosmic break from the cosmic heavy lifting. So, let's embark on a cosmic mission of mindful cosmic eating and regular cosmic movement to keep our cosmic weight in check.

Lastly, let's not forget the cosmic power of good cosmic sleep. A cosmic night of quality cosmic sleep is like a cosmic restoration for our joints. It's like hitting the cosmic reset button, allowing our joints to rejuvenate and repair. So, let's create a cosmic sleep sanctuary, complete with cosmic comfortable pillows, cosmic soothing music, and a cosmic cozy atmosphere that lulls us into the cosmic land of dreams.

Remember, lifestyle factors are like cosmic companions on our joint health journey. With the right cosmic choices, we can empower ourselves to make cosmic lifestyle changes that benefit our joints and overall well-being. So, let's fuel our bodies with cosmic nourishment, keep our joints cosmic moving, manage cosmic stress, maintain a healthy cosmic weight, and embrace the cosmic power of a good cosmic night's sleep. Together, we can rock the cosmic dance floor of life with healthy, happy joints!

# Co-existing conditions

Ah, the cosmic connections between arthritis and co-existing conditions. It's like a celestial dance of intertwined health challenges, a remix of cosmic complexities. Let's explore this cosmic collaboration and shed some light on the cosmic relationships between arthritis and other co-existing conditions.

First up on our cosmic playlist is the dynamic duo of arthritis and cardiovascular disease. They're like two cosmic buddies who often go hand in hand. The cosmic inflammation caused by arthritis can have cosmic repercussions on the heart and blood vessels. So, it's important to keep a cosmic eye on our cardiovascular health by practicing cosmic heart-healthy habits like regular cosmic exercise and cosmic mindful eating.

Next, we have the cosmic collaboration of arthritis and diabetes. They're like two cosmic partners in mischief, challenging our cosmic balance. Arthritis can make cosmic diabetes management a bit more challenging, as physical limitations and cosmic pain can interfere with cosmic exercise and cosmic glucose control. But fear not, cosmic warriors! With the guidance of cosmic healthcare professionals and cosmic lifestyle adjustments, we can navigate this cosmic partnership with cosmic finesse.

And let's not forget about the cosmic connection between arthritis and mental health. They're like two cosmic buddies who sometimes share the same cosmic roller coaster ride. Chronic cosmic pain and physical limitations can take a toll on our cosmic emotional well-being. It's important to address both the cosmic physical and cosmic mental aspects of our health by seeking cosmic support from mental health professionals, practicing cosmic self-care, and finding cosmic coping strategies that work for us.

Now, let's talk about the cosmic connection between arthritis and obesity. They're like two cosmic friends who can exacerbate each other's cosmic challenges. Excess cosmic weight puts extra cosmic pressure on our joints, increasing the risk of cosmic arthritis. On the flip side, cosmic arthritis pain can make cosmic exercise more challenging, contributing to cosmic weight gain. It's a cosmic catch-22, but with cosmic determination and cosmic support, we can break free from this cosmic cycle and achieve a cosmic balance.

Another cosmic duo worth mentioning is arthritis and osteoporosis. They're like two cosmic companions who weaken the cosmic foundations of our cosmic skeletal system. Arthritis-related inflammation and cosmic medications can accelerate cosmic bone loss, increasing the risk of cosmic fractures. So, it's important to focus on cosmic bone health through cosmic calcium-rich foods, cosmic vitamin D, and cosmic weight-bearing exercises to keep our cosmic skeletal system strong.

Last but not least, we have the cosmic connection between arthritis and gastrointestinal disorders. They're like two cosmic buddies who sometimes create cosmic chaos in our digestive system. Certain cosmic medications used to manage arthritis can have cosmic side effects on the gastrointestinal tract, causing cosmic discomfort. It's essential to communicate openly with cosmic healthcare providers about any cosmic gastrointestinal symptoms and find cosmic strategies to manage both cosmic arthritis and cosmic digestive health.

In the cosmic tapestry of our health, these co-existing conditions add complexity to our cosmic journey. But fear not, cosmic adventurers! With the right cosmic support, cosmic healthcare professionals, and cosmic self-care practices, we can navigate this cosmic constellation of challenges and live a fulfilling cosmic life.

Remember, we're all cosmic warriors on this cosmic journey, and even amidst the cosmic complexities, there's always room for a little humor to lighten our cosmic load. So, let's embrace the cosmic connections, seek cosmic support, and dance through the cosmic challenges with grace and a smile on our faces. Together, we can rock the cosmic dance floor of health and well-being!

# Diagnosing Arthritis

Ah, the quest for cosmic diagnosis! Join me on this cosmic journey as we unravel the mysteries of diagnosing arthritis. Grab your cosmic magnifying glass and let's dive in!

Diagnosing arthritis requires a cosmic collaboration between you, your cosmic healthcare provider, and a sprinkle of cosmic medical tests. It's like a cosmic game of clue, where we search for cosmic evidence to reveal the true cosmic culprit behind your cosmic joint pain.

First, your cosmic healthcare provider will embark on a cosmic exploration of your cosmic symptoms and medical history. They'll ask you cosmic questions about the location and nature of your cosmic pain, any cosmic swelling or stiffness, and how these cosmic symptoms impact your cosmic daily life. They might also inquire about any cosmic family history of arthritis or other cosmic autoimmune conditions. So, get ready to share your cosmic story with them, and don't forget to bring your cosmic sense of humor along!

Next, your cosmic healthcare provider might unleash their cosmic superpower—the physical examination. They'll carefully examine your cosmic joints, checking for cosmic tenderness, cosmic swelling, cosmic range of motion, and any cosmic signs of inflammation. They may even perform cosmic maneuvers and ask you to perform cosmic movements to assess your cosmic joint function. It's like a cosmic dance of joint assessment, where they observe your cosmic moves and determine if there are any cosmic red flags.

But wait, the cosmic adventure doesn't end there! Your cosmic healthcare provider might decide to call upon the cosmic forces of medical tests to gather cosmic evidence. Cosmic blood tests can be your cosmic sidekick, helping detect cosmic markers of inflammation and specific cosmic antibodies associated with certain types of arthritis. Imaging cosmic technologies like X-rays, cosmic MRIs, or cosmic ultrasound can provide cosmic glimpses into your cosmic joints, revealing any cosmic signs of damage, cosmic bone spurs, or cosmic joint space narrowing. It's like cosmic peering through a cosmic telescope to unlock the cosmic secrets hidden within your cosmic joints.

Remember, the diagnostic journey can be a cosmic puzzle, and sometimes it takes time to connect all the cosmic pieces. But fear not, cosmic detectives! With patience and cosmic collaboration, we can unveil the truth behind your cosmic joint pain.

Once the cosmic puzzle is solved and a diagnosis is made, it's time to embark on a cosmic treatment plan. Your cosmic healthcare provider will guide you through cosmic options like cosmic medications, cosmic physical therapy, cosmic assistive devices, and cosmic lifestyle modifications. It's like a cosmic toolkit filled with strategies to help you manage your cosmic symptoms and reclaim your cosmic quality of life.

So, embrace the cosmic journey of diagnosis, armed with your cosmic sense of humor and cosmic curiosity. Be an active cosmic participant in the process, asking questions, sharing concerns, and providing cosmic feedback. Remember, you are the protagonist of your cosmic health story, and together with your cosmic healthcare provider, you can navigate the twists and turns of arthritis diagnosis.

In this cosmic dance of diagnosis, humor can be our cosmic ally. It lightens the cosmic mood, eases cosmic tension, and reminds us to find joy even amidst the cosmic challenges. So, let's embark on this cosmic adventure with a smile on our faces and a cosmic determination in our hearts. Together, we can unlock the cosmic secrets of arthritis and pave the way for a cosmic journey towards better health and cosmic well-being!

# The diagnostic process for arthritis

Welcome to the cosmic diagnostic journey of arthritis! Buckle up and prepare for a cosmic adventure as we delve into the diagnostic process for this cosmic condition. Grab your cosmic stethoscope and let's begin!

The diagnostic process for arthritis is like navigating a cosmic maze. Your cosmic healthcare provider will embark on a cosmic exploration of your symptoms, medical history, and perform cosmic tests to unravel the cosmic truth behind your joint discomfort.

First, you'll share your cosmic tale of woe with your cosmic healthcare provider. They'll listen attentively as you describe your cosmic joint pain, stiffness, and any cosmic swelling or redness. Be prepared to provide cosmic details about the affected joints, the duration and intensity of symptoms, and how they impact your cosmic daily activities. Remember, a touch of humor can lighten the cosmic mood and make the journey more enjoyable!

Next, your cosmic healthcare provider will perform a cosmic physical examination. They'll press and prod your cosmic joints, observing for cosmic signs of inflammation, tenderness, and limited cosmic range of motion. This is when you might feel like a cosmic superhero being evaluated for your cosmic powers. Don't worry, it's just a cosmic way for your healthcare provider to gather clues about the cosmic condition lurking within your joints.

But wait, the cosmic adventure doesn't end there! Your cosmic healthcare provider might call upon the cosmic forces of medical tests. Cosmic blood tests can detect cosmic markers of inflammation, such as elevated levels of C-reactive protein or erythrocyte sedimentation rate. These tests are like cosmic detectives searching for evidence of cosmic mischief in your body.

In addition to blood tests, cosmic imaging techniques can provide cosmic insights into your joints. X-rays can reveal cosmic joint damage, cosmic bone spurs, or cosmic joint space narrowing. Magnetic resonance imaging (MRI) and ultrasound can capture cosmic images of your joints, uncovering signs of cosmic inflammation or cosmic joint abnormalities. It's like peering through a cosmic kaleidoscope to see what lies beneath the cosmic surface.

The diagnostic process for arthritis often involves ruling out other cosmic conditions that mimic its symptoms. Your cosmic healthcare provider will make sure there are no cosmic imposters trying to steal the spotlight. This might include ruling out cosmic infections, cosmic autoimmune disorders, or cosmic other systemic diseases. It's like a cosmic game of hide-and-seek, where we eliminate cosmic contenders one by one.

Sometimes, the diagnostic journey for arthritis can be a cosmic puzzle. It requires patience, collaboration, and cosmic persistence to piece together the cosmic clues. Your cosmic healthcare provider may consult with cosmic specialists, such as rheumatologists, to ensure an accurate cosmic diagnosis. Remember, teamwork makes the cosmic dream work!

Once the cosmic puzzle is solved, a diagnosis is made, and the cosmic villain (arthritis) is unmasked, you can embark on a cosmic treatment plan tailored to your needs. Cosmic medications, cosmic physical therapy, cosmic lifestyle modifications, and cosmic support can help you manage your symptoms and improve your cosmic quality of life.

So, let the cosmic diagnostic process guide you to answers and relief. Embrace the journey with curiosity, humor, and an open mind. Remember, you are the protagonist in this cosmic story, and with the cosmic collaboration between you and your healthcare provider, you can conquer the cosmic challenges of arthritis and reclaim your cosmic vitality!

# Common assessment tools and tests

Welcome to the realm of common assessment tools and tests for arthritis! Get ready to dive into the cosmic world of diagnostics and discover the tools that help unlock the secrets of this enigmatic condition. Prepare for a journey filled with cosmic knowledge and a dash of humor!

One of the most commonly used assessment tools in the realm of arthritis is the cosmic questionnaire. It's like a cosmic survey that helps your cosmic healthcare provider gather information about your symptoms, their duration, and the impact they have on your cosmic daily life. It's a bit like filling out a cosmic personality quiz, but instead, you're providing cosmic insights into your joint discomfort.

But wait, there's more! Your cosmic healthcare provider may call upon the cosmic powers of blood tests. These tests can measure cosmic markers of inflammation in your body, such as cosmic C-reactive protein (CRP) and cosmic erythrocyte sedimentation rate (ESR). It's like peering into the cosmic depths of your bloodstream to identify any cosmic signs of mischief.

Another cosmic tool in the diagnostic arsenal is cosmic imaging. X-rays are commonly used to visualize cosmic joint damage, cosmic bone spurs, and cosmic joint space narrowing. It's like taking cosmic snapshots of your joints to uncover hidden cosmic clues. Magnetic resonance imaging (MRI) is another powerful cosmic tool that can provide detailed cosmic images of your joints, revealing cosmic inflammation or cosmic structural abnormalities.

In some cases, a cosmic joint fluid analysis might be requested. This procedure involves extracting a small amount of cosmic fluid from an affected joint and examining it under the cosmic microscope. It's like a cosmic chemistry experiment, where the composition of the fluid can provide cosmic insights into the cosmic condition of your joints.

Now, let's not forget about cosmic joint aspiration. This is when your cosmic healthcare provider uses a cosmic needle and syringe to remove cosmic fluid from a swollen joint. It's like a cosmic version of deflating a balloon to relieve the cosmic pressure. The extracted cosmic fluid can be sent for cosmic laboratory testing to identify any cosmic signs of infection or crystal formation.

Cosmic bone density tests, such as dual-energy X-ray absorptiometry (DXA), are often used to assess cosmic bone health. These tests can determine if you're at risk of cosmic osteoporosis, a condition that can accompany certain forms of arthritis. It's like measuring the cosmic strength of your bones and ensuring they're not playing cosmic Jenga with your joint stability.

Last but not least, your cosmic healthcare provider might call upon the cosmic expertise of a cosmic specialist, such as a rheumatologist. These cosmic specialists are skilled in evaluating the cosmic puzzle of arthritis and may perform additional cosmic assessments, such as cosmic musculoskeletal ultrasound or cosmic joint scintigraphy.

Remember, these cosmic assessment tools and tests serve as valuable cosmic allies in the battle against arthritis. They help your cosmic healthcare provider gather cosmic information, make an accurate cosmic diagnosis, and guide the cosmic treatment plan that best suits your cosmic needs.

So, embrace the cosmic journey of assessments and tests, armed with a sense of curiosity and a sprinkle of humor. Together with your cosmic healthcare team, you'll unlock the cosmic secrets of arthritis and embark on a path towards cosmic wellness!

# Consulting with healthcare providers

Welcome to the cosmic realm of consulting with healthcare providers for arthritis! In this cosmic journey, you'll discover the importance of seeking cosmic guidance from healthcare professionals and how they can be your cosmic allies in managing arthritis. So, grab your cosmic compass and let's embark on this informative and slightly humorous expedition!

When it comes to navigating the vast cosmos of arthritis, consulting with healthcare providers is like having a cosmic GPS system. They have the knowledge and expertise to guide you through the twists and turns of this cosmic condition. Whether it's your cosmic primary care physician or a cosmic specialist like a rheumatologist, these cosmic healthcare professionals are here to help.

But what can you expect during a cosmic consultation? Well, first, be prepared to share your cosmic story. Your healthcare provider will want to know about your cosmic symptoms, their duration, and any factors that worsen or improve them. So, be ready to describe your joint discomfort and its impact on your cosmic daily activities. Remember, the more cosmic details you provide, the better your healthcare provider can understand your cosmic journey.

Next, brace yourself for a cosmic examination. Your healthcare provider may want to get a hands-on cosmic experience of your joints. They might gently probe and manipulate them to assess for cosmic tenderness, swelling, or limited range of motion. Don't worry, they won't summon any cosmic surprises like pulling a rabbit out of a hat, but they may uncover cosmic clues about your arthritis.

Sometimes, additional cosmic tests may be required. Your healthcare provider may order blood tests to measure cosmic markers of inflammation or to rule out other cosmic conditions. They may also request cosmic imaging studies, like X-rays or MRIs, to visualize your cosmic joints and assess for any cosmic abnormalities. These cosmic tests are like peering through a cosmic telescope to get a clearer view of the cosmic universe inside your body.

During your cosmic consultation, it's essential to be an active participant. Ask questions, seek cosmic clarity, and don't be afraid to share any cosmic concerns or uncertainties. Remember, your healthcare provider is there to guide and support you on your cosmic journey.

In addition to your healthcare provider, consider the cosmic benefits of multidisciplinary teams. These teams may include cosmic specialists like physical therapists, occupational therapists, and cosmic dieticians. Each member brings a unique cosmic perspective and skill set to help manage your arthritis. So, don't hesitate to tap into the cosmic expertise of these cosmic professionals. They're like a cosmic Avengers team, but instead of fighting villains, they're fighting arthritis.

Lastly, don't forget the cosmic power of communication. Keep your healthcare provider informed about any changes in your cosmic symptoms, cosmic treatment effectiveness, or any cosmic challenges you face. Be an active cosmic communicator, and together with your healthcare team, you can navigate the cosmic seas of arthritis.

So, as you embark on your cosmic consultations, remember that your healthcare providers are there to be your cosmic guides. With their cosmic expertise and your cosmic collaboration, you'll be equipped to face the challenges of arthritis head-on. Trust the process, embrace the cosmic consultations, and let the cosmic journey towards managing arthritis begin!

# Medication and Arthritis

Welcome to the marvelous world of medication and arthritis! In this journey, we will explore the various cosmic remedies that can help alleviate arthritis symptoms and bring some cosmic relief to your joints. So, grab your cosmic pillbox and get ready for a cosmic adventure filled with information and a sprinkle of humor.

When it comes to managing arthritis, medications can be like cosmic superheroes, fighting off pain, inflammation, and discomfort. Nonsteroidal anti-inflammatory drugs (NSAIDs) are like the Avengers of arthritis medication. They work by reducing inflammation and relieving pain, allowing you to conquer your cosmic activities with less joint discomfort. Just remember, while they can save the day, it's important to use them responsibly and follow your healthcare provider's cosmic guidance.

But NSAIDs are not the only cosmic warriors in the battle against arthritis. Disease-modifying antirheumatic drugs (DMARDs) are like the cosmic Justice League. They target the underlying cosmic mechanisms of arthritis, slowing down its progression and preserving cosmic joint function. These cosmic medications are often used for types of arthritis like rheumatoid arthritis and psoriatic arthritis. They may take some time to show their full cosmic effects, but when they do, you'll feel like a cosmic superhero yourself.

Biologic response modifiers are the cosmic X-Men of arthritis medications. These advanced cosmic treatments are specifically designed to target and block specific cosmic molecules involved in the inflammation process. They can be highly effective in managing certain types of arthritis, such as rheumatoid arthritis and psoriatic arthritis. Think of them as cosmic mutations that bring balance to the cosmic forces causing inflammation in your joints.

Corticosteroids, on the other hand, are like the cosmic magicians of arthritis medications. They have the power to swiftly reduce inflammation and provide immediate relief, but they should be used sparingly and under the cosmic guidance of your healthcare provider. While they can work wonders, their long-term use may come with cosmic side effects, so they're best suited for short-term use in specific cosmic situations.

As you embark on your cosmic medication journey, remember the importance of cosmic communication. Share your cosmic concerns, cosmic medication history, and any cosmic side effects you experience with your healthcare provider. They can adjust your cosmic treatment plan accordingly and help find the best cosmic medication regimen for you.

It's worth noting that medication is not the only cosmic tool in managing arthritis. Lifestyle changes and cosmic self-care play a vital role in cosmic arthritis management. Exercise is like a cosmic workout for your joints, strengthening them and improving flexibility. A cosmic healthy diet can provide the cosmic nutrients your joints need to thrive. And don't forget the cosmic power of rest and relaxation to recharge your cosmic energy.

In conclusion, medication is a cosmic ally in the fight against arthritis. From NSAIDs to DMARDs and biologics, these cosmic remedies can provide much-needed relief and help you regain control over your cosmic joints. Remember, cosmic communication with your healthcare provider is key, and incorporating lifestyle changes will complement the cosmic effects of medication. So, embrace the cosmic power of medication, stay in tune with your cosmic body, and let the cosmic battle against arthritis begin!

# Overview of arthritis medications

Welcome to the wonderful world of arthritis medications, where we'll explore the cosmic pharmacy of options available to help you conquer your arthritis symptoms. So, fasten your seatbelts and prepare for a cosmic journey through the galaxy of arthritis medications, accompanied by a sprinkle of humor.

First on our cosmic list is nonsteroidal anti-inflammatory drugs (NSAIDs), the superheroes of arthritis relief. These cosmic medications help tame inflammation and ease joint pain, allowing you to move with less cosmic discomfort. They're like the cosmic cool kids at the party, always ready to fight off pain and inflammation. Just remember, like any cosmic hero, they have their side effects, so use them responsibly and follow the guidance of your healthcare provider.

Next up, we have disease-modifying antirheumatic drugs (DMARDs), the cosmic agents of change in the battle against arthritis. These cosmic medications work by targeting the cosmic forces behind arthritis and slowing down its progression. They're like the cosmic architects, building a better joint future for you. DMARDs are commonly used for rheumatoid arthritis and other inflammatory types of arthritis. So, let them work their cosmic magic and pave the way to a brighter joint tomorrow.

Biologic response modifiers are the cosmic shape-shifters of arthritis medications. These advanced cosmic treatments target specific cosmic molecules involved in the inflammation process. They're like the cosmic chameleons, adapting to your cosmic needs and modulating the cosmic chaos in your joints. Biologics are often used for conditions like rheumatoid arthritis and psoriatic arthritis, and their cosmic effects can be truly transformational.

Corticosteroids, on the other hand, are like the cosmic firefighters, swiftly extinguishing the flames of inflammation. These cosmic medications provide rapid relief and can be incredibly effective, but they come with their cosmic side effects. Think of them as the cosmic firefighters who save the day but may leave a little water damage behind. They're best used in moderation and under the cosmic guidance of your healthcare provider.

Sometimes, to tackle arthritis, you need a cosmic team effort. Combination therapy involves using different types of arthritis medications together to maximize their cosmic benefits. It's like forming an Avengers-like cosmic alliance to combat your arthritis symptoms. Your healthcare provider will create a cosmic treatment plan tailored to your needs, combining different medications to create a cosmic synergy.

But let's not forget the cosmic power of self-care and lifestyle changes in managing arthritis. While medications play a crucial role, exercise, cosmic nutrition, stress management, and cosmic self-care can enhance their cosmic effects. So, lace up your cosmic sneakers, embrace a cosmic rainbow of fruits and vegetables, find your cosmic zen, and let the cosmic synergy of medication and self-care work its magic.

In conclusion, the cosmic pharmacy of arthritis medications offers a wide range of options to help you navigate the challenges of arthritis. NSAIDs, DMARDs, biologics, corticosteroids, and combination therapy form the cosmic arsenal against arthritis, each with its own cosmic superpowers and considerations. Remember to consult with your healthcare provider to find the right cosmic combination for your specific needs. And don't forget the cosmic value of self-care and lifestyle changes in achieving optimal cosmic joint health. So, grab your cosmic cape, trust in the power of medication and self-care, and conquer the cosmic challenges of arthritis with confidence!

# How medications work to treat arthritis

Welcome to the enchanting world of arthritis medications, where science and magic come together to combat the mighty arthritis. Get ready to dive into the secrets of how these medications work their cosmic wonders, all while enjoying a sprinkle of humor along the way.

Let's start with nonsteroidal anti-inflammatory drugs (NSAIDs), the superheroes of arthritis relief. These cosmic medications work by blocking certain enzymes that contribute to inflammation, just like a cosmic shield protecting your joints from the forces of pain and swelling. They're like the cosmic firefighters, extinguishing the flames of inflammation and bringing peace to your joints.

Next up, we have disease-modifying antirheumatic drugs (DMARDs), the cosmic architects of arthritis treatment. These marvelous medications work behind the scenes, altering the cosmic landscape of your immune system to slow down the progression of arthritis. They're like the cosmic city planners, designing a future where your joints thrive and flourish. So, let them work their cosmic magic and build a solid foundation for joint health.

Biologic response modifiers, on the other hand, are like the cosmic spies infiltrating the realm of arthritis. These cosmic medications target specific molecules in your immune system, disrupting the cosmic communication between cells and dampening the inflammatory response. They're the secret agents fighting the forces of arthritis from within, like a cosmic espionage mission to restore balance in your joints.

Corticosteroids, the cosmic magicians, possess the power to quickly alleviate inflammation and pain. These medications mimic the effects of natural hormones produced by your body, like a cosmic illusionist creating a temporary relief from arthritis symptoms. But beware, their cosmic tricks come with a price, as long-term use may have some side effects. So, let the cosmic magic work its wonders, but with caution.

Sometimes, a combination of medications is needed to conquer arthritis. Like a cosmic team of superheroes, these medications join forces to tackle arthritis from multiple angles. They work together in harmony, each with its unique cosmic powers, to create a cosmic synergy of relief. It's like assembling the Avengers of arthritis treatment, where each medication plays its role in the battle against pain and inflammation.

But let's not forget the importance of self-care in conjunction with medication. Exercise, cosmic nutrition, and lifestyle adjustments act as cosmic sidekicks, supporting the effectiveness of medications. They're like the trusty companions on your cosmic journey to better joint health, working hand in hand with medication to optimize your cosmic results.

In conclusion, arthritis medications work their cosmic wonders by targeting inflammation, modifying the immune system, and providing relief from pain and swelling. NSAIDs, DMARDs, biologics, corticosteroids, and combination therapy each play a unique role in the cosmic battle against arthritis. Remember to consult with your healthcare provider to find the right cosmic combination for your specific needs. And don't forget the cosmic power of self-care and lifestyle adjustments in enhancing the efficacy of medication. So, embrace the magic of arthritis medications and let them be your cosmic allies in the fight against arthritis!

# Common side effects and risks

Welcome to the realm of arthritis treatment, where medications strive to bring relief and cosmic balance to your joints. While these medications work their magic, it's important to be aware of their potential side effects and risks. Fear not, for we shall explore them with a dash of humor and ensure you're well-informed.

Like cosmic travelers on a grand adventure, arthritis medications can occasionally come with some cosmic side effects. Nonsteroidal anti-inflammatory drugs (NSAIDs) may cause gastrointestinal issues, such as cosmic stomach upset or heartburn. But fear not, brave adventurer, for taking these medications with food can help calm the cosmic storm in your belly.

Disease-modifying antirheumatic drugs (DMARDs) may weaken your cosmic immune system, increasing the risk of infections. Consider it a temporary vulnerability, like a superhero without their shield. But fret not, for your healthcare provider will monitor you closely, and with proper precautions, you can conquer both arthritis and the cosmic common cold.

Biologic response modifiers, the cosmic heroes of targeted therapy, may bring forth cosmic allergic reactions. Picture it as a cosmic game of hide and seek, where your immune system seeks out these cosmic agents and decides whether to embrace them or declare them intruders. Stay vigilant, and should you encounter any cosmic reactions, seek the guidance of your healthcare provider.

Corticosteroids, the cosmic magicians, may dazzle with their swift relief, but prolonged use can lead to cosmic side effects. They can cause weight gain, moon-shaped faces, and even cosmic mood swings. Think of it as a magical potion with a time limit, to be used judiciously and with the guidance of your healthcare provider. Remember, laughter is the best cosmic mood stabilizer!

Combining multiple medications may amplify the cosmic side effects. It's like mixing various magical potions in a cosmic cauldron, with the potential for unexpected results. But fear not, for your healthcare provider will carefully craft the cosmic concoction, considering the potential side effects and balancing them with the benefits. Think of them as cosmic alchemists creating the perfect blend for your joint health.

Now, let's delve into the realm of risks. Arthritis medications can sometimes impact the cosmic balance of your body. NSAIDs may elevate blood pressure and increase the risk of cosmic heart attacks and cosmic strokes. But worry not, cosmic warrior, for your healthcare provider will monitor your cosmic vital signs and help keep your cardiovascular system in harmony.

DMARDs and biologic response modifiers may suppress your cosmic immune system, making you more susceptible to infections. But fret not, for with proper precautions and guidance from your healthcare provider, you can navigate this cosmic vulnerability and keep infections at bay.

Cosmic vigilance is necessary when using corticosteroids, as prolonged use can lead to cosmic osteoporosis, elevated blood sugar levels, and even cosmic cataracts. But worry not, for your healthcare provider will monitor your cosmic health and take steps to minimize these risks.

In conclusion, while arthritis medications can bring cosmic relief, it's essential to be aware of their potential side effects and risks. Stay in close communication with your healthcare provider, as they are your cosmic guide through this journey. Remember, humor and knowledge are your cosmic shields, protecting you from the unknown. Together, we shall embrace the cosmic adventure of arthritis treatment, armed with understanding and a sprinkle of humor.

# Non-Medication Approaches to Arthritis Treatment

Welcome, fellow adventurers, to the realm of non-medication approaches to arthritis treatment. While the cosmic forces of medication battle arthritis on one front, there are other strategies that can lend a helping hand. Join me as we explore these alternative paths to relief, with a touch of humor to lighten the cosmic load.

Exercise, the cosmic elixir for the body and mind, takes center stage in our journey. Engaging in regular physical activity can help strengthen the muscles surrounding your joints, like cosmic bodyguards protecting your precious orbs. From yoga to cosmic dance-offs in the living room, find activities that bring joy and movement to your cosmic existence.

Behold, the cosmic power of weight management! Shedding excess pounds can lighten the burden on your joints and reduce the cosmic strain of arthritis. Think of it as shedding unnecessary cosmic baggage, paving the way for a smoother journey. But remember, even cosmic superheroes need a little indulgence every now and then.

The art of heat and cold therapy, a cosmic dance between temperature extremes, can soothe your aching joints. Heat, like a warm cosmic hug, helps relax your muscles and ease stiffness. Cold, on the other hand, acts as a cosmic ice bath, reducing inflammation and numbing cosmic pain. Experiment with both and find the perfect cosmic balance for your unique needs.

Splish, splash, we're taking a cosmic bath! Aquatic therapy, a delightful rendezvous with water, provides a low-impact environment for exercise. Imagine yourself floating weightlessly, the cosmic weight of arthritis temporarily lifted. Just be sure to resist the temptation to become a cosmic mermaid during therapy sessions.

The cosmic power of acupuncture, an ancient art form, may provide relief for arthritis symptoms. Tiny cosmic needles strategically placed along your body's energy pathways can help restore balance and harmony. It's like cosmic acupuncture targeting the cosmic villains of pain and inflammation. But fret not, for the cosmic needles are quite gentle and may even leave you feeling as light as a cosmic feather.

Meditation and mindfulness, the cosmic practices of finding peace within, can also play a role in arthritis management. By focusing your cosmic awareness on the present moment, you can transcend the cosmic pain and find inner calm. Imagine yourself floating among the cosmic stars, your arthritis woes drifting away like distant galaxies.

Dietary cosmic exploration awaits! Some studies suggest that certain foods, like cosmic omega-3 fatty acids and antioxidant-rich fruits and vegetables, may have anti-inflammatory properties. Incorporate these cosmic delights into your diet, knowing that each bite brings you closer to cosmic equilibrium.

In conclusion, non-medication approaches to arthritis treatment offer cosmic alternatives to complement traditional therapies. Embrace the cosmic adventure of exercise, weight management, heat and cold therapy, aquatic escapades, acupuncture, meditation, mindful cosmic journeys, and dietary exploration. Remember, humor and curiosity are your cosmic companions on this path. Consult with your healthcare provider to craft a cosmic treatment plan that suits your individual needs. Together, let us navigate the cosmic realm of arthritis management with open hearts and cosmic resilience.

# Physical therapy for arthritis

Greetings, brave adventurers! Today, we embark on a quest to explore the cosmic realm of physical therapy for arthritis. It's time to unlock the secrets of movement, laughter, and healing. So gather your cosmic energy and let's dive in!

Physical therapy, the cosmic art of movement, is a powerful ally in the battle against arthritis. Skilled physical therapists will guide you through a cosmic journey of exercises and techniques tailored to your unique needs. Together, you'll uncover the cosmic dance of mobility and strength, defeating the cosmic villains of pain and stiffness.

Ah, the wonders of cosmic exercise! Under the guidance of your physical therapist, you'll engage in a variety of activities designed to improve your joint flexibility, cosmic endurance, and cosmic balance. From gentle cosmic stretches to cosmic resistance training, each movement is a step closer to reclaiming your cosmic vitality. Just be sure to unleash your inner superhero during these sessions, as it adds a touch of cosmic flair.

Fear not, for physical therapy sessions are not all cosmic sweat and tears. Laughter, the cosmic medicine, is often part of the journey. Physical therapists have an uncanny ability to infuse humor into their cosmic routines, turning each session into a joyful cosmic adventure. So prepare your cosmic funny bone and get ready to giggle your way to cosmic wellness.

Did you know that physical therapy is not limited to the cosmic walls of a clinic? Your physical therapist can equip you with cosmic exercises to practice at home. These cosmic homework assignments are your secret weapons in the fight against arthritis. But remember, consistency is key, so make sure to channel your cosmic determination and follow your therapist's instructions diligently.

Now, let's talk about the cosmic wonders of manual therapy. Picture yourself lying on a cosmic table, as your physical therapist applies cosmic techniques to mobilize your joints and release cosmic tension. It's like receiving a cosmic massage from a skilled celestial being. Just be prepared for the occasional cosmic crack, as your therapist works their cosmic magic.

Balance training, the cosmic tightrope act, plays a crucial role in physical therapy for arthritis. Through cosmic exercises and challenges, you'll enhance your cosmic stability and reduce the risk of cosmic falls. Think of it as preparing for a cosmic acrobatic performance, where your body gracefully defies the cosmic forces of imbalance.

As you progress in your cosmic physical therapy journey, you may discover the cosmic benefits of assistive devices. From cosmic braces to walking aids, these tools can provide additional support and relieve cosmic stress on your joints. Embrace them as cosmic companions on your path to cosmic wellness.

In conclusion, physical therapy for arthritis is a cosmic adventure filled with movement, laughter, and healing. It empowers you to regain control of your cosmic body, overcome limitations, and find joy in motion. Remember, your physical therapist is your cosmic guide, so trust in their expertise and embrace the cosmic journey they have planned for you. Together, you'll navigate the twists and turns of arthritis, forging a cosmic path towards strength, flexibility, and cosmic well-being.

# Occupational therapy for arthritis

Welcome, adventurers, to the realm of occupational therapy for arthritis! Prepare to embark on a journey that combines creativity, practicality, and a touch of humor to conquer the challenges of daily life with arthritis.

Occupational therapy is not about finding a new cosmic occupation but rather about optimizing your ability to perform the activities that matter most to you. Think of it as your cosmic toolkit, filled with strategies and adaptations to overcome the cosmic obstacles arthritis throws your way.

One of the cosmic wonders of occupational therapy is its focus on cosmic adaptations. Your occupational therapist, a master of creativity, will uncover cosmic solutions to make everyday tasks more manageable. From cosmic gadgets that ease your grip to ergonomic cosmic modifications in your environment, they'll transform your cosmic realm into an arthritis-friendly space.

Remember, cosmic heroes, there's no need to be shy about seeking cosmic assistance. Occupational therapy embraces the concept of cosmic teamwork. Your therapist may introduce you to cosmic aids such as jar openers, reachers, or even cosmic adaptive utensils. These tools are not just practical but also cosmic conversation starters at your next dinner party.

But wait, there's more! Occupational therapy also delves into the cosmic depths of energy conservation. Arthritis can drain your cosmic energy, making even simple tasks feel like cosmic quests. Fear not, for your occupational therapist will teach you the cosmic art of pacing and prioritizing. They'll guide you in breaking down tasks, allocating energy wisely, and avoiding the cosmic temptation to conquer Mount Everest in a single day.

Cosmic creativity shines in occupational therapy's approach to joint protection. Your therapist will teach you cosmic techniques to minimize stress on your cosmic joints while performing daily activities. It's like being a cosmic ninja, gracefully dodging cosmic pain and preserving your cosmic joints for future adventures.

Now, let's talk about the cosmic dance of activity modification. Your occupational therapist will work with you to adapt activities to your unique abilities and limitations. It's all about finding cosmic alternatives that allow you to continue engaging in activities you enjoy. So, if knitting your cosmic masterpiece becomes a challenge, fear not! Your therapist might introduce you to adaptive knitting tools that keep your cosmic creativity flowing.

Fatigue management is another cosmic skill occupational therapy addresses. Arthritis can sometimes leave you feeling like you've battled cosmic dragons all day long. Your therapist will help you develop cosmic strategies to conserve energy and balance activity with rest. Remember, cosmic warriors, even superheroes need their cosmic nap time!

Lastly, let's not forget about the cosmic realm of mental well-being. Occupational therapy recognizes the cosmic connection between mind and body. Your therapist may incorporate cosmic relaxation techniques, stress management strategies, and mindfulness exercises to cultivate cosmic serenity amidst the chaos of arthritis.

In conclusion, occupational therapy for arthritis is a cosmic adventure that equips you with the tools, adaptations, and strategies to conquer daily challenges with creativity and humor. It empowers you to maintain independence, engage in activities that bring you joy, and find cosmic balance in the face of arthritis. So, embrace your occupational therapist as your cosmic ally, and together, embark on a quest to reclaim your cosmic kingdom of functionality and cosmic well-being.

# Natural remedies and alternative therapies

Welcome, fellow explorers, to the realm of natural remedies and alternative therapies for arthritis. Prepare to embark on a journey where ancient wisdom meets modern science, sprinkled with a dash of humor, to tame the arthritis beast.

While the cosmic world of natural remedies and alternative therapies may seem like uncharted territory, it has been traversed by many brave souls before us. Let's delve into some cosmic strategies that have captured the attention of both cosmic adventurers and scientists alike.

First on our cosmic quest is the celestial herb known as turmeric. This golden spice, with its cosmic anti-inflammatory properties, has been revered for centuries. So, spice up your cosmic cuisine with a sprinkle of turmeric and let its magic dance through your cosmic joints.

Next, we encounter the cosmic wonders of acupuncture. This ancient cosmic art involves the strategic placement of cosmic needles to stimulate energy flow and cosmic healing. Imagine yourself as a cosmic porcupine, embracing the cosmic balance of yin and yang.

But wait, there's more! The cosmic realm of meditation and mindfulness beckons us. Dive into the cosmic depths of relaxation and tranquility, leaving stress behind like a distant cosmic memory. Find your cosmic Zen through practices like deep breathing, guided imagery, or even cosmic laughter yoga. Remember, even the cosmos itself takes time to recharge.

Another celestial gem in our arsenal is omega-3 fatty acids. These cosmic superheroes, found in fatty fish like salmon, possess anti-inflammatory powers that can help soothe the cosmic flames of arthritis. So, grab your cosmic fishing rod and set sail on a delicious cosmic voyage.

The cosmic practice of yoga invites us to stretch, strengthen, and find harmony in our cosmic bodies. Explore cosmic poses that enhance flexibility, improve cosmic balance, and promote a cosmic sense of well-being. Embrace your inner cosmic warrior and flow through the cosmic sequences.

Let's not forget the cosmic power of heat and cold therapy. Like cosmic magicians, these modalities offer relief to inflamed joints. Soak in a cosmic hot bath or apply a cosmic ice pack to tame the cosmic fire within.

As we journey deeper, we stumble upon the cosmic realm of herbal supplements. From cosmic ginger to cosmic devil's claw, these botanical warriors have been used for centuries to combat cosmic inflammation. However, tread carefully in this cosmic terrain and consult with a cosmic healthcare provider to ensure cosmic safety.

Now, let's not overlook the cosmic healing powers of laughter. Yes, you heard it right! Laughter is cosmic medicine. It releases cosmic endorphins, reduces stress, and brings cosmic joy to your soul. So, gather your cosmic companions, watch a cosmic comedy, and let the laughter ripple through the cosmos.

Lastly, we encounter the cosmic world of essential oils. From cosmic lavender to cosmic peppermint, these aromatic wonders offer cosmic relief to tired joints and muscles. Anoint yourself with cosmic scents and let them transport you to a cosmic oasis of tranquility.

In conclusion, the cosmic realm of natural remedies and alternative therapies offers a myriad of options to complement conventional treatments for arthritis. While they may not work for everyone, their cosmic potential is worth exploring. Remember to consult with your cosmic healthcare provider before embarking on any cosmic journey. So, embrace the cosmic wonders that nature and ancient wisdom provide, and may your path to cosmic well-being be filled with laughter, peace, and cosmic relief.

# Managing Arthritis Pain

Welcome to the cosmic realm of managing arthritis pain, where we embark on a quest to tame the unruly beast known as pain. Join me on this enlightening journey as we explore strategies to conquer pain and restore cosmic harmony to our lives.

First and foremost, let's unleash the power of heat and cold therapy. Imagine yourself as a cosmic chef, cooking up a delightful recipe for pain relief. Apply a cosmic heating pad or indulge in a cosmic ice pack to soothe your cosmic joints. Find the perfect balance between hot and cold, like a cosmic master chef creating a culinary masterpiece.

Now, let's embrace the cosmic wonders of exercise. Engaging in regular cosmic movement can be a potent weapon against pain. But fear not, we're not talking about running marathons or becoming cosmic bodybuilders. Find activities that bring you cosmic joy, like cosmic dancing, gentle yoga, or even a cosmic stroll in nature. Remember, laughter is cosmic exercise too, so let your inner cosmic comedian shine.

Speaking of laughter, it's time to unleash its cosmic healing powers. Laughter releases cosmic endorphins, our very own cosmic painkillers. So, gather your cosmic comedy club and enjoy a cosmic laughter-filled evening. Remember, laughter is contagious, so spread it like cosmic wildfire and watch pain retreat into the cosmic shadows.

Let's not forget the cosmic art of relaxation and stress management. Picture yourself floating on a cosmic cloud, surrounded by tranquility and serenity. Engage in cosmic practices like deep breathing, meditation, or cosmic mindfulness. Embrace your inner cosmic Zen master and let stress melt away like a cosmic ice cream cone on a hot summer day.

In the cosmic world of nutrition, we have some cosmic allies too. Embrace a cosmic diet rich in anti-inflammatory foods. Load up on cosmic fruits and vegetables, whole grains, and cosmic omega-3 fatty acids from sources like cosmic fish or chia seeds. Be the cosmic chef of your own kitchen, creating cosmic meals that nourish your body and combat pain.

Now, let's tap into the cosmic powers of technology. Explore cosmic gadgets like cosmic pain trackers or cosmic meditation apps. Let your smartphone become your cosmic companion on this journey, offering cosmic reminders, cosmic relaxation exercises, and even cosmic motivational messages. Embrace the cosmic synergy between technology and pain management.

The cosmic realm of natural remedies also extends to topical treatments. From cosmic creams to cosmic salves, these cosmic concoctions can provide temporary cosmic relief. So, imagine yourself as a cosmic alchemist, concocting the perfect blend of cosmic ingredients to soothe your cosmic joints.

Last but not least, let's dive into the cosmic world of support networks. Surround yourself with cosmic beings who understand and empathize with your cosmic pain. Join cosmic support groups, engage in cosmic conversations, and share cosmic stories. The cosmic bond that forms will bring cosmic comfort and make you feel less alone on your cosmic journey.

In conclusion, managing arthritis pain is a cosmic adventure that requires a multidimensional approach. Embrace the power of heat and cold, explore cosmic movement, laughter, relaxation techniques, and a cosmic diet. Utilize the cosmic benefits of technology, natural remedies, and the support of cosmic companions. Remember, pain may be a formidable foe, but armed with knowledge, humor, and a cosmic spirit, you can reclaim control over your cosmic well-being. So, let the cosmic quest begin, and may pain be no match for your cosmic resilience.

# Strategies for managing arthritis pain

Welcome to the world of arthritis pain management, where we embark on a quest to conquer the mighty beast called pain. Join me on this enlightening journey as we explore strategies to tame the pain and restore balance to our lives.

First, let's dive into the cosmic world of heat and cold therapy. Imagine yourself as a master of elemental forces, harnessing the power of hot and cold to soothe your aching joints. Apply a warm cosmic compress or indulge in an icy cosmic sensation to find the perfect balance between heat and cold. You'll feel like a cosmic wizard, conjuring relief from the depths of discomfort.

Next, let's explore the cosmic wonders of exercise. Engaging in regular cosmic movement can be a powerful weapon against pain. But don't worry, we're not suggesting you join a cosmic marathon or become a cosmic weightlifter. Find activities that bring you cosmic joy, like cosmic dancing or gentle yoga. You'll be a pain-fighting superhero, leaping over obstacles with cosmic grace.

Laughter is truly cosmic medicine. It releases cosmic endorphins, the body's natural pain relievers. So, gather your cosmic comedy club and enjoy a cosmic laughter session. Let your inner cosmic comedian shine, and watch pain retreat like a cosmic coward in the face of humor.

Relaxation techniques are another cosmic tool in your arsenal. Picture yourself floating on a cosmic cloud, surrounded by tranquility and peace. Engage in cosmic practices like deep breathing, meditation, or cosmic mindfulness. Let stress melt away like an ice cream cone on a cosmic summer day, leaving you refreshed and pain-free.

In the cosmic realm of nutrition, we have some cosmic allies too. Embrace a cosmic diet rich in anti-inflammatory foods. Load up on cosmic fruits and vegetables, whole grains, and cosmic omega-3 fatty acids from sources like cosmic fish or chia seeds. Be the cosmic chef of your own kitchen, creating meals that nourish your body and combat pain.

Technology can be a cosmic sidekick in pain management. Explore cosmic gadgets like cosmic pain trackers or cosmic meditation apps. Let your smartphone become your cosmic companion, offering cosmic reminders, relaxation exercises, and even cosmic motivational messages. Embrace the cosmic synergy between technology and pain relief.

Topical treatments can also provide cosmic relief. From cosmic creams to cosmic ointments, these cosmic concoctions can offer temporary respite. Imagine yourself as a cosmic alchemist, concocting the perfect blend of cosmic ingredients to soothe your cosmic joints.

Last but not least, surround yourself with cosmic allies in the form of support networks. Join cosmic support groups, engage in cosmic conversations, and share cosmic stories. The cosmic bond that forms will bring cosmic comfort and make you feel less alone on your cosmic journey.

In conclusion, managing arthritis pain is a cosmic adventure that requires a multidimensional approach. Embrace the power of heat and cold, explore cosmic movement and laughter, and practice relaxation techniques. Nourish your body with a cosmic diet, utilize technology as a cosmic aid, and consider topical treatments. Surround yourself with cosmic companions who understand and support you. Together, we can conquer the pain and reclaim control over our cosmic well-being. So, let the cosmic quest begin, and may pain be no match for our cosmic resilience.

# Exercise and physical activity for arthritis

Welcome to the world of arthritis and physical activity, where we embark on a journey of movement, strength, and cosmic joint health. Join me on this enlightening adventure as we explore the benefits of exercise for arthritis and discover how to make physical activity a joyful part of our lives.

When it comes to arthritis, it's easy to picture our joints as grumpy old cosmic beings, resistant to movement. But fear not, for exercise is like a cosmic superhero that can help loosen up those creaky joints and improve our overall cosmic well-being.

First, let's talk about the cosmic benefits of exercise for arthritis. Regular cosmic physical activity can help reduce joint pain and stiffness, improve flexibility and range of motion, and strengthen the cosmic muscles around our joints. It's like giving our cosmic joints a cosmic spa treatment, complete with soothing massages and cosmic rejuvenation.

But we're not talking about running a cosmic marathon or doing cosmic acrobatics here. The key is to find cosmic activities that suit our individual needs and preferences. It could be cosmic walking, cosmic swimming, or even cosmic dancing. The important thing is to move our bodies and have cosmic fun while doing it.

Now, let's sprinkle some cosmic humor into our exercise routine. Picture yourself as a cosmic superhero, ready to conquer the world of arthritis with your superpowers of movement. Don your cosmic exercise gear, complete with a cape if you so desire, and let the cosmic adventures begin. Laugh at your cosmic quirks and embrace the joy of cosmic activity.

Warm up your cosmic muscles before diving into exercise. Imagine yourself as a cosmic ballerina, gracefully performing cosmic stretches to prepare your body for action. Stretching helps improve flexibility, reduce the risk of injury, and increase cosmic flow throughout your body. Embrace your cosmic gracefulness and let the cosmic movements flow.

Now, it's time for the main event: the cosmic exercise routine. Start with low-impact cosmic exercises that are gentle on your joints. Cosmic cycling, cosmic yoga, or cosmic tai chi are excellent choices. These activities can help strengthen cosmic muscles, improve cosmic balance, and give your joints the cosmic love they deserve.

Don't forget to listen to your cosmic body. If a particular cosmic exercise causes pain or discomfort, modify it or try something else. It's all about finding the cosmic sweet spot that works best for you.

Incorporate cosmic strength training into your routine. Use cosmic resistance bands or cosmic light weights to strengthen cosmic muscles around your joints. Think of it as cosmic weightlifting, but with a playful twist. Remember, cosmic strength training doesn't mean bulging muscles. It's about cosmic empowerment and building cosmic resilience.

Finally, cool down your cosmic body after exercise. Imagine yourself as a cosmic yogi, gracefully transitioning from activity to relaxation. Cosmic stretching and deep breathing help your body recover and prevent cosmic soreness. Embrace the cosmic serenity that comes with the cool-down phase.

In conclusion, exercise and physical activity are cosmic allies in the battle against arthritis. They can help reduce pain, improve flexibility, and strengthen cosmic muscles. Embrace the cosmic joy of movement, whether it's walking, swimming, dancing, or engaging in other activities that make you feel alive. Laugh at your cosmic quirks and find humor in your cosmic superhero journey. Remember, you have the power to create your own cosmic exercise routine and make it a delightful part of your cosmic life. So, let's put on our cosmic sneakers and embark on this cosmic adventure of cosmic joint health. Together, we can conquer arthritis and embrace the cosmic joy of movement.

# Heat and cold therapy for arthritis

Welcome to the world of hot and cold, where we explore the magical powers of temperature in soothing our arthritis woes. Join me on this informative journey as we dive into the cosmic realms of heat and cold therapy for arthritis.

Let's start with heat therapy, our cosmic cozy blanket for achy joints. Imagine yourself enveloped in a warm cosmic embrace, as heat gently eases your cosmic discomfort. Applying heat to arthritic joints helps increase blood flow, relax cosmic muscles, and reduce cosmic pain. It's like a cosmic spa day for your joints, complete with warm towels and soothing cosmic music.

Now, picture yourself as a cosmic ice queen or king, ready to embrace the chill of cold therapy. Cold therapy, in the form of ice packs or cold compresses, can help reduce inflammation and numb cosmic pain. It's like a refreshing cosmic breeze on a hot summer day, cooling down those inflamed joints and giving you a moment of cosmic relief.

But before we delve deeper into the cosmic realms of temperature, let's sprinkle a little humor to lighten the cosmic mood. Imagine your arthritic joints as cosmic adventurers, embarking on a quest to find the perfect temperature balance. Will they choose the warm and cozy path or venture into the icy wonders of cold therapy? Let the cosmic journey begin!

Now, let's explore when to use each cosmic therapy. Heat therapy is excellent for soothing chronic arthritis pain and stiffness. It's like a cosmic hug for your joints, providing comfort and relaxation. Apply heat to the affected area for around 20 minutes at a time, using a warm towel, heating pad, or even a cosmic hot water bottle. Just be careful not to overheat and turn into a cosmic fireball!

On the other hand, cold therapy works wonders for acute arthritis pain and swelling. Imagine yourself as a cosmic Eskimo, embracing the icy coldness to calm down inflammation. Apply a cold pack or wrap ice cubes in a towel and place it on the affected area for about 15 minutes. But remember, don't keep the cold therapy on for too long, or you might turn into a cosmic ice sculpture!

Experiment with cosmic temperature variations to find your cosmic sweet spot. Some individuals find relief by alternating between hot and cold therapy. It's like a cosmic dance of temperature, keeping your joints on their toes. Just remember to listen to your cosmic body and adjust accordingly.

Don't forget to use cosmic caution when applying heat or cold therapy. Protect your cosmic skin by using a barrier, such as a towel, between the temperature source and your skin. And if you have sensory issues or reduced sensitivity, be mindful of the temperature to avoid cosmic surprises.

Lastly, embrace the cosmic relaxation that comes with heat and cold therapy. Picture yourself in a cosmic oasis, with warm and cold sensations melting away your arthritis troubles. Find comfort in the cosmic embrace of temperature, knowing that you have a cosmic tool to soothe your achy joints whenever needed.

In conclusion, heat and cold therapy are cosmic allies in the battle against arthritis. They provide relief, reduce inflammation, and offer a cosmic respite for your joints. Embrace the cosmic adventures of finding the right temperature balance and let the warmth or chill work its magic. Remember to approach temperature therapy with cosmic humor and creativity, turning your arthritis journey into a cosmic exploration of comfort and relief. So, get ready to embrace the cosmic heat or chill and discover the cosmic wonders of heat and cold therapy for arthritis.

# Managing Arthritis Inflammation

Welcome to the fiery world of arthritis inflammation! In this informative and humor-filled journey, we'll explore strategies for managing the flames of inflammation that often accompany arthritis. So, grab your cosmic fire extinguisher and let's dive in!

Imagine your joints as cosmic firefighters, bravely battling the flames of inflammation. But fear not, for we have an arsenal of cosmic tools to keep the fire under control. Let's sprinkle some humor along the way to lighten the cosmic mood and bring a smile to your inflamed joints.

The first strategy in our cosmic toolkit is medication. It's like a superhero cape for your joints, swooping in to save the day. Nonsteroidal anti-inflammatory drugs (NSAIDs) such as ibuprofen and naproxen can help tame the cosmic flames of inflammation. Just be sure to consult your cosmic doctor before using any medication, as they will guide you on the cosmic dosage and potential side effects.

Next up, we have the cosmic diet. Imagine your plate as a cosmic battleground, where you choose foods that either fuel the flames or douse them. Omega-3 fatty acids found in fish, flaxseeds, and walnuts have anti-inflammatory properties, making them your cosmic allies. On the other hand, cosmic villains like saturated fats and processed sugars can fan the flames of inflammation. So, choose your cosmic meals wisely, and remember, a salad a day keeps the inflammation away!

Let's move on to the cosmic power of exercise. It's like a cosmic firefighter training camp for your joints, building strength and resilience. Low-impact exercises such as swimming, yoga, and cosmic dancing can help reduce inflammation and improve joint function. But beware, avoid high-impact activities like cosmic skydiving or wrestling cosmic bears, as they may aggravate inflammation. Safety first, cosmic adventurers!

Now, picture yourself in a cosmic chill-out zone, where stress melts away like cosmic ice cream. Stress can fuel inflammation, so finding ways to manage it is crucial. Explore cosmic stress management techniques like meditation, deep breathing, or even cosmic laughter therapy. Remember, laughter is the best cosmic medicine, and it can extinguish the flames of stress-induced inflammation.

Next on our cosmic journey is cosmic cold therapy. Just as ice cubes soothe a cosmic sunburn, applying cold packs or using cold compresses can help calm inflammation in your joints. It's like a refreshing cosmic plunge into an icy pool on a scorching summer day. But remember, don't turn into a cosmic ice sculpture! Limit cold therapy sessions to around 15 minutes at a time and always use a barrier, like a towel, to protect your cosmic skin.

Last but not least, we have the cosmic power of rest and relaxation. Picture yourself as a cosmic sloth, lounging in a cosmic hammock, and letting your joints take a well-deserved break. Rest is crucial for managing inflammation, as it allows your cosmic firefighters to recharge and regroup. Get plenty of cosmic beauty sleep and find cosmic activities that promote relaxation, like cosmic bubble baths or stargazing.

In conclusion, managing arthritis inflammation requires a cosmic toolkit of strategies. From medication to diet, exercise to stress management, cold therapy to rest, you have the power to keep the cosmic flames of inflammation under control. Embrace the cosmic humor along the way, as laughter truly is the cosmic medicine. So, equip yourself with your cosmic firefighter gear and face the flames of inflammation with confidence. Remember, you have the power to keep your cosmic joints cool, calm, and collected.

# Strategies for managing arthritis inflammation

Welcome to the cosmic battle against arthritis inflammation! In this informative and humor-infused adventure, we'll explore strategies to conquer the fiery enemy that often accompanies arthritis. Get ready to arm yourself with knowledge and a cosmic sense of humor as we embark on this journey together.

The first strategy in our cosmic arsenal is medication. Think of it as your trusty sidekick in the fight against inflammation. Nonsteroidal anti-inflammatory drugs (NSAIDs) such as ibuprofen and naproxen can help calm the cosmic flames and provide relief. But remember, always consult your cosmic doctor to ensure you're using the right cosmic dosage and minimize potential side effects.

Next up, we have the cosmic power of nutrition. Imagine your plate as a cosmic battleground, with each food choice having the potential to fuel or extinguish the flames of inflammation. Embrace cosmic superheroes like fruits, vegetables, whole grains, and lean proteins that have anti-inflammatory properties. But watch out for the cosmic villains—processed foods, sugary treats, and trans fats—these can stoke the cosmic fire. Choose your cosmic meals wisely and be a nutrition superhero!

Now, let's put on our cosmic sneakers and dive into the world of exercise. Engaging in regular physical activity can be a cosmic game-changer in managing arthritis inflammation. Low-impact exercises like swimming, cycling, or cosmic tai chi can help strengthen your cosmic joints while keeping inflammation at bay. Just be sure to warm up your cosmic muscles before diving into any activity and listen to your cosmic body's signals to avoid overdoing it.

In addition to exercise, the cosmic power of stress management cannot be underestimated. Stress is like fuel to the cosmic flames of inflammation, so finding ways to keep it in check is vital. Embrace cosmic stress-busting techniques like deep breathing exercises, yoga, or even a cosmic dance party in your living room. Remember, laughter is the cosmic stress-buster supreme, so sprinkle your cosmic days with humor and surround yourself with positive cosmic energy.

Now, let's explore the cosmic realm of heat therapy. Just as warmth soothes the cosmic soul, applying heat to inflamed joints can provide much-needed relief. Consider using warm towels, heat packs, or taking cosmic baths to ease the cosmic inflammation. Just be mindful of not turning yourself into a cosmic marshmallow—moderation is key.

Lastly, let's tap into the cosmic power of rest and relaxation. Adequate sleep and rest are essential in managing inflammation. Imagine yourself floating on a cosmic cloud, allowing your cosmic body and joints to rejuvenate. Establish a cosmic bedtime routine, create a calm cosmic environment, and bid farewell to cosmic distractions that might interfere with your cosmic sleep.

In conclusion, managing arthritis inflammation requires a cosmic combination of strategies. Medication, nutrition, exercise, stress management, heat therapy, and rest are your cosmic allies in the battle against inflammation. Embrace the power of these strategies and infuse them with your cosmic sense of humor. Remember, you're the hero of your cosmic story, and with the right tools and a sprinkle of laughter, you can conquer the fiery enemy of arthritis inflammation. So, gear up, embrace the cosmic adventure, and unleash your inner superhero to keep the flames at bay.

# Anti-inflammatory diet and supplements

Welcome to the delicious and anti-inflammatory world of cosmic nutrition! In this informative and humor-infused journey, we'll explore the power of food and supplements in the battle against arthritis inflammation. Get ready to tantalize your taste buds and embrace your inner cosmic chef as we dive into this culinary adventure.

Let's start with the cosmic heroes of the anti-inflammatory diet. Picture them as a team of culinary Avengers, ready to save the day. Fruits and vegetables lead the charge, providing a cosmic arsenal of antioxidants and phytochemicals that combat inflammation. Berries, leafy greens, and colorful cosmic vegetables are your cosmic allies. Embrace their vibrant colors and make your plate a work of art.

Next up, we have the mighty Omega-3 fatty acids, the cosmic guardians of inflammation. These cosmic superheroes can be found in fatty fish like salmon, mackerel, and sardines. They wield their anti-inflammatory power by reducing the production of cosmic villains called cytokines. So, reel in these fishy cosmic heroes and let them swim into your cosmic diet.

Speaking of cosmic villains, let's talk about trans fats and their nefarious plans to stoke the cosmic flames of inflammation. These sneaky culprits hide in processed snacks, fast food, and cosmic pastries. Show them no mercy, and banish them from your cosmic pantry. Opt for healthy cosmic fats instead, like avocados, nuts, and cosmic olive oil, which possess anti-inflammatory properties.

But wait, there's more to this cosmic nutrition adventure! Supplements can be the cosmic boost you need to combat inflammation. Start with the cosmic duo of glucosamine and chondroitin, known for their joint-protective powers. These cosmic companions can help reduce inflammation and improve joint health. Just make sure to consult your cosmic doctor before adding them to your cosmic routine.

Turmeric, the golden spice of cosmic healing, deserves a special mention. Its active compound, curcumin, has potent anti-inflammatory properties. Sprinkle it on your cosmic meals or whip up a cosmic turmeric latte for a flavorful and anti-inflammatory cosmic treat. Just remember, a little goes a long way!

Probiotics, the cosmic gut guardians, also play a role in managing inflammation. These friendly bacteria help maintain a cosmic balance in your gut, which can influence inflammation levels. Add some cosmic yogurt or fermented foods to your cosmic diet to support your gut health and keep inflammation at bay.

Now, let's sprinkle a little cosmic humor into our journey. Imagine a cosmic spice rack filled with laughter, joy, and positivity. Studies show that laughter can reduce inflammation and promote overall well-being. So, let's infuse our cosmic nutrition adventure with a generous sprinkle of humor and embrace the healing power of laughter.

In conclusion, the anti-inflammatory diet and supplements are your cosmic allies in the battle against arthritis inflammation. Embrace the cosmic power of fruits, vegetables, Omega-3 fatty acids, and cosmic spices like turmeric. Bid farewell to cosmic villains like trans fats and welcome healthy cosmic fats into your life. Consider supplements like glucosamine, chondroitin, and probiotics to enhance your cosmic arsenal. And remember, laughter is the cosmic spice that adds flavor and joy to your anti-inflammatory cosmic journey. So, grab your cosmic apron, whip up some delicious anti-inflammatory cosmic meals, and let your taste buds and joints rejoice in this cosmic culinary adventure.

# Stress reduction techniques for arthritis

Welcome to the world of stress-busting strategies, where we'll explore how to keep arthritis and stress at bay through cosmic relaxation techniques. Picture yourself floating on a cloud of tranquility as we journey through this informative and humor-infused exploration.

First, let's talk about the cosmic power of deep breathing. Take a moment to inhale peace and exhale stress. Deep breathing activates the cosmic relaxation response, reducing stress hormones and promoting a sense of calm. So, take a cosmic breath and let your worries float away like tiny cosmic bubbles.

Now, let's add a dash of cosmic humor to our stress-reduction recipe. Laughter is the cosmic medicine that can lighten your mood and melt away stress. Watch a cosmic comedy show, read a funny book, or share a cosmic joke with a friend. Remember, laughter is the cosmic glue that holds our cosmic well-being together.

Meditation, the cosmic zen master, is another powerful tool in our stress-fighting arsenal. Find a quiet cosmic corner, close your eyes, and let your mind wander among the cosmic stars. Meditation helps calm the cosmic storm within, allowing you to find inner peace amidst the chaos of life. Embrace your inner cosmic guru and let the stress melt away.

Exercise, the cosmic energizer, not only keeps our bodies fit but also helps alleviate stress. Engaging in cosmic activities like walking, yoga, or dancing releases endorphins, the cosmic feel-good hormones. So, put on your cosmic sneakers and dance away your worries or stretch your cosmic limbs with some cosmic yoga poses.

Next, let's add a cosmic touch to our stress reduction journey with aromatherapy. Essential oils like lavender, chamomile, and eucalyptus possess cosmic calming properties. Create a cosmic oasis in your home by diffusing these soothing scents or adding a few drops to your cosmic bath. Allow the cosmic aroma to transport you to a stress-free cosmic paradise.

The cosmic power of music cannot be underestimated. Tune in to your favorite cosmic playlist and let the celestial melodies transport you to a cosmic state of relaxation. Whether it's classical, jazz, or cosmic rock, find the cosmic rhythm that resonates with your soul and let the stress fade away.

Massage, the cosmic tension whisperer, is a luxurious way to release stress and tension. Treat yourself to a cosmic massage or enlist a cosmic partner to give you a soothing cosmic rubdown. Feel the cosmic knots in your muscles unwind as you surrender to the cosmic touch.

Last but not least, the power of connection cannot be overlooked. Surround yourself with cosmic friends and loved ones who bring joy and support into your life. Share your cosmic journey with them, and let their cosmic presence be a source of comfort and stress relief. Remember, we are all connected in this cosmic dance of life.

In conclusion, stress reduction techniques are the cosmic keys to managing arthritis and promoting overall well-being. Embrace the power of deep breathing, laughter, meditation, exercise, aromatherapy, music, massage, and cosmic connections. Allow these cosmic techniques to transport you to a stress-free cosmic realm where arthritis and stress fade away. So, take a cosmic break, indulge in relaxation, and let the cosmic calm wash over you. Your body and mind will thank you as you embark on this cosmic journey to a stress-free and harmonious life.

# Arthritis and Exercise

Welcome to the world of exercise, where we'll dive into the marvelous relationship between arthritis and physical activity. Get ready to embark on an informative and humor-filled journey that will inspire you to get moving and conquer arthritis with a smile.

When it comes to arthritis, exercise might sound like an oxymoron. But fear not, because movement is actually your secret weapon against the cosmic forces of joint pain and stiffness. Think of exercise as your trusty sidekick in the battle against arthritis. Together, you'll form a dynamic duo that will keep you on your toes (literally!).

So, what can exercise do for you in the cosmic fight against arthritis? Well, for starters, it strengthens the cosmic muscles around your joints, providing them with extra support. It's like building a fortress of strength to protect your joints from the cosmic invaders of pain and inflammation.

But wait, there's more! Exercise also helps improve your cosmic range of motion, allowing you to bend, stretch, and twist with ease. It's like giving your joints a cosmic yoga class, teaching them to be flexible and nimble. Who knew arthritis could be so cosmic?

Now, let's add a sprinkle of humor to our exercise routine. Picture yourself in a cosmic aerobics class, wearing your brightest cosmic leggings and grooving to the beat of the cosmic music. Dance away your arthritis woes and laugh at the cosmic irony that you're defying the odds with every move.

But exercise doesn't have to be all cosmic dance parties. Low-impact activities like swimming and cycling are gentle on your joints while still giving them a cosmic workout. Dive into the cosmic pool or hop on a cosmic bike and let the cosmic endorphins flow. It's like a cosmic party for your joints!

Strength training, the cosmic muscle builder, is another vital component of an arthritis-friendly exercise routine. Grab those cosmic dumbbells and challenge your muscles to new heights. As your cosmic strength increases, your joints will rejoice, knowing they have a cosmic army of muscles to rely on.

Don't forget the cosmic power of stretching and flexibility exercises. Yoga, Pilates, or cosmic stretching routines can help keep your joints supple and mobile. Embrace your cosmic inner yogi and find your zen amidst the cosmic chaos of arthritis.

Remember, when it comes to exercise and arthritis, consistency is key. Aim for at least 30 minutes of moderate-intensity exercise most days of the week. Break it down into cosmic bite-sized chunks if needed and listen to your cosmic body. If pain or discomfort persists, consult with your cosmic healthcare provider for guidance.

In conclusion, exercise is the cosmic elixir for arthritis. It strengthens your muscles, improves flexibility, and keeps your joints happy and healthy. So, put on your cosmic sneakers, dance, swim, cycle, lift weights, and stretch. Embrace the cosmic humor of defying the odds and reclaim your cosmic mobility. Arthritis may knock on your cosmic door, but with exercise as your cosmic ally, you'll show it who's boss. Get moving, embrace the cosmic power of exercise, and let arthritis know that you're not backing down without a fight.

# Benefits of exercise for arthritis

Get ready to discover the extraordinary benefits of exercise for arthritis in this informative and humor-filled chapter. Brace yourself for a cosmic journey where we'll explore the wonders of physical activity and its profound impact on arthritis.

When it comes to arthritis, exercise is like a cosmic superhero that swoops in to save the day. It has a myriad of benefits that can make a world of difference in managing arthritis symptoms. Think of exercise as your trusty sidekick, ready to fight off joint pain and stiffness with a dose of cosmic humor.

One of the incredible benefits of exercise is its ability to strengthen the cosmic muscles surrounding your joints. By engaging in regular physical activity, you're essentially building an army of strong cosmic warriors that support and protect your joints. It's like having a secret cosmic weapon against the forces of arthritis!

But that's not all. Exercise also helps to improve your cosmic range of motion. It's like giving your joints a cosmic yoga class, teaching them to be flexible and mobile. Picture yourself in a yoga pose, defying gravity and defying the limitations of arthritis. Who said arthritis couldn't be a little cosmic?

Now, let's sprinkle some humor into our exercise routine. Imagine yourself in a cosmic aerobics class, wearing the most colorful leggings and dancing to the beat of cosmic music. Laugh at the cosmic irony as you defy arthritis with every move, showing it that you won't be held back.

Exercise doesn't have to be all cosmic dance parties, though. Low-impact activities like swimming and cycling can be gentle on your joints while still providing a cosmic workout. Dive into the pool or hop on your cosmic bike and let the endorphins flow. It's like a cosmic party for your joints!

Strength training, the cosmic muscle builder, is another incredible benefit of exercise for arthritis. It helps to increase muscle strength and endurance, providing even more support to your joints. It's like giving your joints a cosmic entourage of muscles to lean on.

Don't underestimate the power of cosmic stretching and flexibility exercises. Yoga, Pilates, or cosmic stretching routines can help improve joint mobility and reduce stiffness. Embrace your inner yogi and find your cosmic zen amidst the challenges of arthritis.

Regular exercise also plays a cosmic role in managing weight and maintaining a healthy body mass index (BMI). Excess weight puts additional strain on your joints, so by engaging in physical activity, you're taking a cosmic step towards relieving that burden.

Additionally, exercise promotes better overall health, boosting your cardiovascular system, and enhancing your cosmic mood. It's like a cosmic cocktail of well-being, leaving you energized, uplifted, and ready to conquer the cosmic challenges of arthritis.

In conclusion, exercise is the cosmic key to unlocking a world of benefits for arthritis. It strengthens your muscles, improves flexibility, manages weight, and enhances overall well-being. So, put on your cosmic sneakers, dance, swim, cycle, lift weights, and stretch. Embrace the cosmic power of exercise and let arthritis know that you're not backing down without a fight. Remember, consult with your healthcare provider before starting any new exercise program and listen to your cosmic body. Get moving, laugh at the cosmic irony, and show arthritis that you're the one in charge.

# Types of exercise for arthritis

Get ready to embark on a cosmic journey through the galaxy of exercise options for arthritis. In this informative and humor-filled chapter, we'll explore the various types of exercises that can help manage arthritis symptoms. Buckle up and prepare for a cosmic adventure that will leave you with a smile on your face.

First up on our cosmic tour is low-impact aerobic exercises. These exercises are like a cosmic dance party for your joints, providing cardiovascular benefits without putting excessive strain on them. Think of it as dancing through the universe with your arthritis as your dance partner. From cosmic walking to water aerobics, these activities will keep your joints moving and your heart pumping.

Next, we encounter the cosmic world of strength training. This type of exercise involves using cosmic resistance, such as dumbbells or resistance bands, to strengthen your cosmic muscles and protect your joints. It's like giving your joints a cosmic bodyguard who won't let arthritis push them around. Remember to start with light weights and gradually increase as your cosmic muscles become stronger.

Flexibility exercises are the cosmic key to maintaining joint mobility and reducing stiffness. Think of them as the cosmic yoga class for your joints. From gentle cosmic stretches to cosmic yoga poses, these exercises will keep your joints limber and ready for any cosmic adventure that comes your way.

Aquatic exercises, such as swimming or water aerobics, offer a cosmic twist to your workout routine. The buoyancy of water reduces the stress on your joints, making it an ideal choice for those with arthritis. It's like experiencing zero gravity while exercising, giving your joints a much-needed break from the pressures of gravity on Earth.

Now, let's dive into the cosmic realm of tai chi and yoga. These mind-body practices focus on gentle movements, deep breathing, and cosmic relaxation. They promote balance, flexibility, and a sense of cosmic peace. It's like finding your cosmic center amidst the challenges of arthritis. Embrace the cosmic flow and let your body and mind find harmony.

For those seeking a cosmic adventure, consider cycling. Whether it's exploring cosmic landscapes on a stationary bike or venturing into the cosmic wilderness on a real one, cycling provides a low-impact cardiovascular workout while minimizing stress on your joints. It's like riding through the galaxy, feeling the cosmic breeze on your face.

Lastly, let's not forget about the cosmic power of walking. It's a simple yet effective exercise that can be enjoyed anywhere, anytime. Lace up your cosmic sneakers and embark on a cosmic stroll. Remember, each step you take is like a cosmic victory against arthritis. Walk at your own pace and enjoy the cosmic scenery along the way.

In conclusion, the universe of exercise options for arthritis is vast and diverse. From low-impact aerobics to strength training, flexibility exercises to aquatic workouts, and cosmic tai chi to cycling and walking, there's a cosmic exercise option for everyone. So, put on your cosmic gear, embrace the cosmic adventures, and let arthritis know that you're ready to conquer the galaxy with your cosmic moves. Remember to consult with your healthcare provider before starting any new exercise program and listen to your cosmic body. Get moving, have fun, and keep exploring the cosmic wonders of exercise for arthritis.

# Building an exercise routine with arthritis

Are you ready to embark on a cosmic journey to build an exercise routine that will conquer arthritis? In this informative chapter, we will explore the key steps to creating an exercise routine that is both effective and enjoyable. Get ready to discover your cosmic workout routine and show arthritis who's boss!

Step one on our cosmic journey is to consult with your healthcare provider. They are the cosmic guides who will provide valuable insights and recommendations based on your specific needs and abilities. Think of them as the navigators of your cosmic exercise journey, steering you in the right direction.

Next, let's set realistic goals. While we may dream of becoming cosmic superheroes, it's important to start with achievable goals. Aim for small, cosmic victories that will gradually build your confidence and momentum. Remember, even cosmic superheroes had to start with baby steps.

Now it's time to choose the cosmic exercises that suit your needs and preferences. There are a plethora of options to choose from, ranging from cosmic swimming to cosmic yoga and everything in between. Find the cosmic activities that bring you joy and make you feel like a cosmic superstar.

To maintain your cosmic routine, consistency is key. Think of it as committing to a cosmic quest and sticking to it. Find a routine that works for you, whether it's exercising at the same cosmic time each day or dedicating specific cosmic days to different activities. Consistency will keep your cosmic momentum going.

Listen to your cosmic body. It's important to find a balance between challenging yourself and taking cosmic rest when needed. Remember, your cosmic body is unique and deserves respect. If you need a cosmic break, take it. Rest, rejuvenate, and come back stronger than ever.

Stay cosmicly motivated. One way to do this is by mixing up your routine. Explore different cosmic exercises, try new cosmic classes, and embrace the cosmic variety. This will keep you excited, engaged, and prevent the cosmic boredom monster from creeping in.

Don't forget about the cosmic power of warm-up and cool-down exercises. They are the cosmic bookends of your workout, preparing your cosmic body for action and helping it recover. It's like cosmic stretching before a cosmic adventure and cooling down after conquering the galaxy.

Embrace the cosmic power of community. Joining cosmic exercise groups or classes can provide support, motivation, and a cosmic sense of belonging. Plus, it's more fun to conquer the galaxy with fellow cosmic warriors by your side.

Lastly, don't let setbacks discourage you. Arthritis may throw cosmic curveballs, but remember that you are a cosmic warrior capable of overcoming challenges. Keep your cosmic sense of humor intact, laugh in the face of adversity, and bounce back stronger than ever.

In conclusion, building an exercise routine with arthritis is like embarking on a cosmic adventure. Consult with your healthcare provider, set realistic goals, choose cosmic exercises that bring you joy, and maintain consistency. Listen to your cosmic body, mix up your routine, warm up and cool down, embrace community, and stay resilient in the face of setbacks. You are a cosmic warrior capable of conquering arthritis and enjoying the cosmic benefits of exercise. So, put on your cosmic cape, grab your cosmic dumbbells, and let the cosmic journey to a healthier, more active life begin! Remember, the universe is your playground, and arthritis doesn't stand a chance against your cosmic determination.

# Arthritis and Diet

Welcome to the cosmic world of arthritis and diet! In this informative chapter, we will explore the relationship between what you eat and arthritis. Get ready to discover how the power of nutrition can help you combat arthritis and lead a cosmic life!

First things first, let's talk about inflammation—the cosmic villain behind arthritis. Certain foods can either fuel or fight inflammation. Think of it as a cosmic battle between the Avengers and Thanos, where your diet is the ultimate weapon. So, it's time to assemble your cosmic team of anti-inflammatory foods.

Let's start with the cosmic superheroes of nutrition—fruits and vegetables. These colorful powerhouses are packed with antioxidants, vitamins, and minerals that have cosmic anti-inflammatory properties. Embrace the cosmic rainbow and fill your plate with cosmic kale, spinach, berries, and all the cosmic goodness nature has to offer.

Next, let's talk about the cosmic wonders of omega-3 fatty acids. These superhero fats can be found in fatty fish like salmon, mackerel, and sardines. They have cosmic anti-inflammatory effects and can help soothe arthritis symptoms. So, grab your cosmic fishing rod and reel in those omega-3s!

Now, it's time to give a cosmic shout-out to the humble whole grains. They are the cosmic energy source that provides complex carbohydrates and fiber, keeping your cosmic body fueled and your digestion cosmicly smooth. Swap refined grains for whole grains like quinoa, brown rice, and cosmic oats.

Don't forget the cosmic power of spices. Turmeric, ginger, and cinnamon are like cosmic wizards fighting inflammation with their magical properties. Sprinkle them in your cosmic dishes and let them work their cosmic charm.

As much as we love cosmic heroes, it's time to talk about the cosmic villains—saturated fats and processed foods. These are the Loki and Ultron of nutrition, contributing to inflammation and worsening arthritis symptoms. Limit cosmic villains like fried foods, processed snacks, and cosmic fast food. Your cosmic body will thank you.

Hydration is crucial in the cosmic battle against arthritis. Water keeps your cosmic joints lubricated and helps flush out toxins. So, grab your cosmic water bottle and stay hydrated throughout the cosmic day.

Now, let's talk about portion control. Just like in the cosmic universe, balance is key. Eating too much of even the healthiest foods can lead to cosmic weight gain, which puts extra stress on your cosmic joints. So, be mindful of your portions and listen to your cosmic body's hunger cues.

Lastly, let's address the cosmic elephant in the room—alcohol and arthritis. While a cosmic toast now and then is perfectly fine, excessive cosmic alcohol consumption can worsen inflammation and interfere with arthritis medications. So, sip your cosmic drinks in moderation.

In conclusion, the cosmic connection between arthritis and diet is like a cosmic dance between superheroes and villains. Embrace the power of anti-inflammatory foods, fill your cosmic plate with fruits, vegetables, whole grains, and omega-3 fatty acids. Spice up your cosmic dishes with turmeric, ginger, and cinnamon. Avoid cosmic villains like saturated fats and processed foods. Stay hydrated, practice portion control, and be mindful of your cosmic alcohol consumption. Remember, nutrition is your cosmic weapon against arthritis. So, grab your cosmic fork and knife, and let the cosmic battle begin!

Disclaimer: The cosmic advice provided in this chapter is for informative purposes only and should not replace professional medical advice. Consult with your healthcare provider or a registered dietitian for personalized cosmic nutrition recommendations. And always remember to maintain your cosmic sense of humor throughout your cosmic journey to a healthier, arthritis-friendly diet.

# The impact of diet on arthritis symptoms

Welcome to the wacky world of diet and arthritis symptoms! In this informative and humor-filled chapter, we'll explore how your food choices can affect those pesky arthritis symptoms. Get ready to embark on a culinary adventure that will make you laugh and learn!

Picture this: you're on a culinary rollercoaster, and every bite you take has the potential to either fuel or soothe your arthritis symptoms. It's like a culinary showdown between your fork and those bothersome symptoms.

Let's start with the pain party crashers—foods that may worsen arthritis symptoms. Just like your neighbor's loud party, these culprits can amplify inflammation and trigger discomfort. Say goodbye to your rowdy neighbors: processed foods, sugary treats, and fried goodies. They may taste heavenly, but they can send your arthritis symptoms through the roof. So, wave them goodbye and invite their healthier alternatives to the party.

Now, let's bring in the arthritis symptom soothers—foods that can help calm the inflammation storm. These are like the superheroes of nutrition, fighting off those pesky symptoms. Say hello to the Avengers of your diet: fruits, vegetables, and whole grains. They are packed with antioxidants and fiber, which have anti-inflammatory properties. So, load up your plate with a colorful array of cosmic veggies and fruits, and enjoy the superpowers of plant-based goodness!

But wait, there's more! Omega-3 fatty acids are the sidekicks you need to tame your arthritis symptoms. Found in fatty fish like salmon, mackerel, and sardines, these healthy fats can help reduce inflammation and give your symptoms a well-deserved break. So, grab your cape and indulge in some cosmic seafood!

We can't forget the cosmic wonders of spices. Turmeric, the superstar of spices, has anti-inflammatory properties that may alleviate arthritis symptoms. Add a dash of turmeric to your cosmic recipes and let it work its magic. And don't forget the other cosmic flavor boosters like ginger, garlic, and cinnamon. They not only add pizzazz to your dishes but also have anti-inflammatory powers.

Now, let's talk about the hydration station. Water is like the cosmic elixir that keeps your joints lubricated and flushes out toxins. It's like a refreshing shower for your cosmic body. So, raise your cosmic water bottle and drink up!

Remember, portion control is like the cosmic DJ that keeps the party in check. Eating too much, even of the healthiest foods, can lead to cosmic weight gain and put extra stress on your joints. So, listen to your cosmic body's cues and practice portion control. Let's keep the party in balance!

In conclusion, your diet can be a powerful ally in managing arthritis symptoms. By choosing foods that are rich in antioxidants, fiber, omega-3 fatty acids, and spices, you can help reduce inflammation and tame those pesky symptoms. So, say goodbye to the pain party crashers like processed foods and sugary treats, and invite the arthritis symptom soothers to the table. And don't forget to stay hydrated and practice portion control to keep the cosmic balance. With a little culinary creativity and a sprinkle of humor, you can conquer those arthritis symptoms one delicious bite at a time!

Disclaimer: The cosmic advice provided in this chapter is for informative purposes only and should not replace professional medical advice. Consult with your healthcare provider or a registered dietitian for personalized dietary recommendations. And always remember to maintain your cosmic sense of humor throughout your culinary journey to manage arthritis symptoms.

# Foods to eat and avoid for arthritis

Welcome to the cosmic kitchen, where we'll uncover the secrets of foods to eat and avoid for arthritis! In this informative and humor-filled chapter, we'll explore the culinary choices that can either soothe or aggravate your arthritis symptoms. Get ready for a gastronomic adventure that will leave you laughing and well-informed!

Let's start with the cosmic superheroes of arthritis-friendly foods. These champions have anti-inflammatory properties that can help ease those nagging symptoms. Say hello to the leafy green warriors like spinach and kale, the berry brigade of blueberries and strawberries, and the nutty avengers such as almonds and walnuts. These foods are rich in antioxidants, vitamins, and minerals that can give your joints a cosmic boost.

Now, let's address the villains of arthritis aggravation—the foods that may trigger inflammation and worsen your symptoms. Imagine them as the sneaky troublemakers lurking in the shadows, ready to sabotage your cosmic joint health. Say goodbye to their mischief: processed foods, sugary snacks, and high-fat delights. While they may seem tempting, they can be like cosmic kryptonite to your joints, so it's best to keep them at bay.

But fear not! We have cosmic substitutes that can satisfy your cravings without wreaking havoc on your joints. Swap those greasy fries with baked sweet potato wedges, trade sugary sodas for sparkling water with a splash of cosmic citrus, and replace processed snacks with cosmic homemade trail mix. These substitutes are not only tasty but also have the power to support your joint health.

In the cosmic spice cabinet, we have some secret weapons to add flavor and fight inflammation. Turmeric, the golden superhero, contains curcumin, which has been studied for its anti-inflammatory properties. So, sprinkle it on your cosmic dishes and let the flavor and benefits bloom. And don't forget about cosmic ginger, known for its potential to reduce inflammation and soothe upset stomachs. It's like a cosmic duo that brings both flavor and relief.

Let's not forget our cosmic friends from the sea—omega-3 fatty acid-rich fish. Salmon, mackerel, and sardines are like cosmic swimmers with a mission to calm inflammation and support joint health. So, reel them in and enjoy their cosmic benefits. If you're not a fan of seafood, fear not! Flaxseeds and chia seeds are cosmic plant-based alternatives that also pack a punch of omega-3 fatty acids.

Now, let's raise our cosmic glasses and toast to hydration! Water is the cosmic elixir that keeps your joints lubricated and flushes out toxins. It's like a cosmic spa treatment for your joints. So, sip on water throughout the day and keep those joints happy and hydrated.

In conclusion, your cosmic culinary choices can play a vital role in managing arthritis symptoms. Embrace the cosmic superheroes like leafy greens, berries, nuts, and omega-3-rich fish, as they can help calm inflammation and support joint health. Bid farewell to the troublemakers of inflammation, such as processed foods and sugary treats. And don't forget to spice up your cosmic dishes with turmeric, ginger, and other flavorful herbs and spices. Stay hydrated with cosmic water and listen to your body's cues to create a cosmic balance in your diet.

Disclaimer: The cosmic advice provided in this chapter is for informative purposes only and should not replace professional medical advice. Consult with your healthcare provider or a registered dietitian for personalized dietary recommendations. And remember, maintaining a cosmic sense of humor throughout your culinary journey will only enhance the cosmic experience of managing arthritis with food!

# Building a healthy eating plan with arthritis

Welcome to the cosmic kitchen, where we'll whip up a healthy eating plan designed specifically for those with arthritis! In this informative and humor-filled chapter, we'll guide you through the cosmic aisles of nutrition, helping you build a meal plan that supports your joint health. Get ready to embark on a cosmic culinary adventure that will leave you both educated and entertained!

First things first, let's talk about the cosmic superheroes of a healthy eating plan for arthritis. These are the nutrient-packed foods that can give your joints the love and care they deserve. Picture them as the cosmic avengers ready to fight inflammation and promote overall well-being. We have the vibrant team of fruits and vegetables, bursting with antioxidants and essential vitamins. Think of them as the cosmic defenders, protecting your joints from harm.

Now, let's bring in the cosmic protein powerhouses to the scene. Lean sources of protein like chicken, fish, tofu, and legumes are like the muscle-bound heroes, providing your body with the building blocks it needs for repair and recovery. They also help maintain a healthy weight, which can reduce stress on your joints. So, invite them to your cosmic feast and let them fuel your joint health.

The cosmic grains and cereals are here to add some cosmic crunch to your healthy eating plan. Whole grains like quinoa, brown rice, and oats are packed with fiber and essential nutrients. They're like the cosmic sidekicks, providing long-lasting energy and supporting your digestive health. So, let them join your cosmic party and add a wholesome touch to your meals.

But what about those cosmic villains that can sabotage your healthy eating plan? They are the sneaky culprits hiding in processed foods, sugary treats, and unhealthy fats. Let's call them the "Junk Food League." They may be tempting, but they can trigger inflammation and worsen arthritis symptoms. So, it's best to keep them at a safe cosmic distance. Remember, even heroes need to avoid the occasional cosmic battle.

Now, let's sprinkle some cosmic flavor into your meals with herbs, spices, and healthy fats. Cosmic herbs like basil, oregano, and rosemary not only add a delightful aroma but also offer anti-inflammatory benefits. They're like the cosmic magicians, turning your dishes into flavorful masterpieces. And don't forget about cosmic healthy fats like avocados, olive oil, and nuts—they're like the cosmic lubricants for your joints, providing essential nutrients and reducing inflammation.

In order to create a cosmic balance in your eating plan, portion control and listening to your body's cues are crucial. Pay attention to your hunger and fullness signals, and practice mindful eating. This will help you build a healthy relationship with food and prevent overeating, which can put extra stress on your joints.

In conclusion, building a healthy eating plan with arthritis is like assembling a cosmic team of nutritional superheroes. Embrace the power of fruits, vegetables, lean proteins, and whole grains while keeping the cosmic villains of processed foods and unhealthy fats at bay. Spice up your cosmic dishes with herbs and healthy fats, and practice portion control and mindful eating. Remember, a healthy eating plan is not about restriction—it's about nourishing your body and supporting your joint health.

Disclaimer: The cosmic advice provided in this chapter is for informative purposes only and should not replace professional medical advice. Consult with your healthcare provider or a registered dietitian for personalized dietary recommendations. And remember, maintaining a cosmic sense of humor throughout your cosmic culinary journey will only enhance the joy of building a healthy eating plan with arthritis!

# Arthritis and Sleep

Welcome to the realm of slumber, where we dive into the cosmic connection between arthritis and sleep. In this enlightening and humor-infused chapter, we'll explore the importance of quality sleep in managing arthritis and unveil some cosmic secrets to help you catch those elusive Z's. So, get ready to embark on a cosmic journey that will leave you both informed and entertained!

When it comes to arthritis, sleep plays a vital role in your overall well-being. It's like the cosmic restoration chamber that allows your body to heal, recharge, and combat the cosmic villains of inflammation and pain. However, arthritis can often disrupt this cosmic harmony, making it challenging to achieve restful slumber.

One of the primary culprits stealing your precious sleep is pain. Arthritis pain can be as stubborn as a cosmic supervillain, causing discomfort and restlessness. To tame this villain, consider incorporating some cosmic bedtime rituals. Experiment with relaxation techniques like deep breathing, gentle stretching, or cosmic meditation to help ease pain and promote a peaceful sleep environment.

Another cosmic enemy of sleep for those with arthritis is joint stiffness. Imagine waking up feeling as rigid as a cosmic statue! To combat this stiffness, a cosmic pre-sleep ritual might involve a warm bath or a gentle cosmic massage. This can help relax your muscles and joints, making it easier to drift off into cosmic dreamland.

But fear not, for the cosmic superheroes of sleep are here to save the day! Establishing a cosmic sleep routine can be the secret weapon to overcoming sleep difficulties caused by arthritis. Set a consistent bedtime and wake-up time to regulate your body's internal cosmic clock. Create a cosmic sleep sanctuary by keeping your bedroom cool, dark, and quiet—just like a cosmic retreat for relaxation.

Now, let's talk about the cosmic sidekicks of sleep—your sleep environment and cosmic sleep posture. Ensure your mattress and pillows provide adequate support for your joints, aligning them in a cosmic dance of comfort. Experiment with different sleeping positions to find the one that minimizes joint pressure and maximizes cosmic relaxation.

Cosmic nutrition also plays a role in promoting restful sleep. Avoid cosmic villains like caffeine and heavy meals close to bedtime, as they can disrupt your cosmic slumber. Instead, opt for cosmic allies like a soothing cup of herbal tea or a cosmic bedtime snack rich in tryptophan, like a cosmic banana.

Lastly, let's not forget the cosmic power of regular exercise in promoting better sleep. Engaging in cosmic activities like walking, swimming, or yoga can help manage arthritis symptoms and contribute to a more restorative sleep. Just make sure to schedule your cosmic workouts earlier in the day to avoid cosmic energy boosts right before bedtime.

In conclusion, understanding the cosmic dance between arthritis and sleep is crucial for managing your condition and improving your quality of life. Embrace cosmic rituals like relaxation techniques, warm baths, and gentle stretching to ease pain and stiffness. Establish a consistent cosmic sleep routine, create a sleep sanctuary, and consider cosmic nutrition and regular exercise as your allies in achieving restful slumber.

Disclaimer: The cosmic advice provided in this chapter is for informational purposes only and should not replace professional medical advice. Consult with your healthcare provider for personalized recommendations tailored to your specific arthritis needs. And remember, maintaining a cosmic sense of humor as you navigate the realm of arthritis and sleep will help you conquer any cosmic sleep challenges that come your way!

# The impact of arthritis on sleep

Welcome to the realm of sleep, where the cosmic battle between arthritis and peaceful slumber unfolds. In this informative yet entertaining chapter, we delve into the impact of arthritis on sleep and unveil the secrets to achieving a restful night's rest. So, buckle up and prepare for a cosmic journey that will leave you both enlightened and amused!

Arthritis, like a mischievous cosmic creature, can wreak havoc on your sleep patterns. The pain and discomfort caused by arthritis can make it challenging to find the cosmic sweet spot of slumber. As if the cosmic forces conspired against you, joint inflammation and stiffness can turn your bed into a battlefield of discomfort.

Picture this cosmic scene: as you attempt to drift off into dreamland, arthritis pain barges in like an uninvited cosmic villain. It disrupts your peaceful cosmic dance of sleep, causing restlessness and frustration. But fear not, for we shall uncover some cosmic secrets to combat these nocturnal disturbances.

One cosmic strategy to minimize the impact of arthritis on sleep is to create a cosmic sleep sanctuary. Optimize your bedroom environment by making it cool, dark, and quiet—a peaceful retreat from the cosmic chaos of the day. Invest in a comfortable mattress and cosmic pillows that provide ample support to your achy joints.

The timing of cosmic activities also plays a role in the impact of arthritis on sleep. Engaging in cosmic exercises earlier in the day, rather than right before bedtime, can help alleviate arthritis symptoms and prevent cosmic energy boosts that may interfere with your cosmic slumber. So, save the energetic cosmic battles for daytime and embrace the tranquility of the night.

Now, let's talk about the cosmic relationship between arthritis and sleep positions. Just like superheroes, certain sleep positions can come to your rescue. Experiment with different cosmic sleep postures to find the one that eases joint pressure and promotes cosmic comfort. It may take a bit of cosmic trial and error, but the effort is worth it for a good night's rest.

Cosmic nutrition also plays a role in the impact of arthritis on sleep. A balanced cosmic diet rich in anti-inflammatory foods can help manage arthritis symptoms and promote better sleep. Incorporate cosmic allies like fruits, vegetables, whole grains, and cosmic omega-3 fatty acids into your meals. Say goodbye to cosmic villains like sugary treats and excessive cosmic caffeine that may disrupt your cosmic slumber.

Lastly, stress reduction techniques can be the cosmic superpowers that combat the impact of arthritis on sleep. Engage in cosmic activities like meditation, deep breathing, or cosmic relaxation exercises before bedtime. These cosmic techniques can help calm your mind and prepare you for a restful journey through the cosmic realm of sleep.

In conclusion, arthritis can be a cosmic disruptor of sleep, but with the right cosmic strategies, you can reclaim your restful slumber. Create a cosmic sleep sanctuary, engage in cosmic exercises at the appropriate times, find cosmic sleep positions that alleviate joint pressure, nourish your body with a cosmic diet, and embrace stress reduction techniques. Remember, humor can be a powerful cosmic force, so maintain a lighthearted approach as you navigate the cosmic dance between arthritis and sleep.

Disclaimer: The cosmic advice provided in this chapter is for informational purposes only and should not replace professional medical advice. Consult with your healthcare provider for personalized recommendations tailored to your specific arthritis needs. And remember, maintaining a cosmic sense of humor as you battle arthritis's impact on sleep will make the journey a little lighter and brighter!

# Strategies for improving sleep with arthritis

Welcome to the cosmic quest for a good night's sleep in the realm of arthritis! In this enlightening and amusing chapter, we will explore strategies for improving sleep while managing the challenges of arthritis. Get ready for a cosmic adventure that will leave you both informed and entertained!

Arthritis, the cosmic nemesis of restful slumber, often disrupts the tranquility of the cosmic realm of sleep. However, fear not, for we shall embark on a cosmic journey to discover strategies that can help you reclaim your cosmic rest.

Firstly, creating a cosmic sleep routine can work wonders for improving sleep with arthritis. Establishing a consistent bedtime and wake-up time sets your cosmic internal clock and signals to your body when it's time for rest. It's like aligning the cosmic stars to create a harmonious sleep pattern.

In the cosmic battle against arthritis-induced sleep disturbances, your cosmic sleep environment plays a crucial role. Transform your cosmic sleep sanctuary into a haven of comfort and tranquility. Invest in a cosmic mattress and pillows that provide optimal support for your joints. Soft cosmic lighting, soothing sounds, and cosmic aromatherapy can create a serene atmosphere conducive to cosmic rest.

The cosmic power of relaxation techniques should not be underestimated. Engaging in cosmic practices like meditation, progressive muscle relaxation, or cosmic visualization before bedtime can calm your mind and prepare you for a peaceful cosmic slumber. Imagine floating among the stars as you let go of cosmic tension and invite cosmic relaxation.

Cosmic sleep positions can also make a cosmic difference when it comes to arthritis and sleep. Experiment with different cosmic sleep postures to find the one that minimizes joint pressure and maximizes cosmic comfort. It's like discovering the perfect cosmic dance move that brings cosmic relief to your achy joints.

Another cosmic strategy is to manage pain and inflammation before bedtime. Cosmic pain management techniques such as applying heat or cold therapy, using topical creams, or taking over-the-counter pain relievers can help alleviate discomfort and promote cosmic sleep. It's like providing a cosmic shield against arthritis's nocturnal disruptions.

Cosmic nutrition can also contribute to better sleep with arthritis. Avoid consuming cosmic stimulants like caffeine close to bedtime, as they can interfere with your cosmic slumber. Instead, indulge in cosmic foods rich in cosmic nutrients, such as cosmic magnesium, cosmic calcium, and cosmic melatonin, which can support a restful cosmic sleep.

Cosmic exercise during the day can prepare your body for a cosmic journey to dreamland. Engage in gentle cosmic exercises, such as cosmic stretching or cosmic yoga, to promote joint flexibility and cosmic relaxation. Remember, it's like warming up for the cosmic adventure of sleep.

Lastly, don't underestimate the power of cosmic comfort aids. Cosmic tools such as supportive cosmic pillows, cosmic compression gloves, or cosmic joint braces can provide extra cosmic relief and enhance your cosmic sleep experience. It's like equipping yourself with cosmic gadgets to navigate the challenges of arthritis during sleep.

In conclusion, by incorporating these cosmic strategies into your sleep routine, you can improve sleep quality while managing arthritis. Establish a cosmic sleep routine, create a cosmic sleep environment, practice relaxation techniques, explore cosmic sleep positions, manage pain and inflammation, consider cosmic nutrition, engage in cosmic exercise, and utilize cosmic comfort aids. Remember, laughter is cosmic medicine, so maintain a cosmic sense of humor as you navigate the cosmic dance between arthritis and sleep.

Disclaimer: The cosmic advice provided in this chapter is for informational purposes only and should not replace professional medical advice. Consult with your healthcare provider for personalized recommendations tailored to your specific arthritis needs. And remember, with the right cosmic strategies, you can achieve a cosmic sleep that rejuvenates both your body and mind!

# Sleep aids and supports for arthritis

Welcome to the world of cosmic sleep aids and supports for arthritis! In this enlightening and amusing chapter, we will explore a variety of cosmic tools and techniques that can help you find sweet cosmic dreams despite the challenges of arthritis. Get ready for a cosmic adventure filled with information and a sprinkle of humor!

When arthritis tries to disrupt your cosmic slumber, sleep aids can come to the rescue. One of the most common cosmic sleep aids for arthritis is a cosmic pillow. These magical pillows are designed to provide cosmic support to your neck and spine, promoting proper alignment and relieving cosmic pressure on your joints. It's like resting your cosmic head on a fluffy cloud of comfort.

If cosmic pillow power alone doesn't do the trick, consider cosmic mattress toppers. These celestial wonders can transform your ordinary mattress into a cosmic haven of cosmic support. They are designed to distribute your cosmic weight evenly and alleviate cosmic pressure on your joints. It's like adding a touch of cosmic magic to your sleeping surface.

Cosmic heat therapy can also be a game-changer in the cosmic battle against arthritis-induced sleep disturbances. Cosmic heating pads or cosmic electric blankets can provide soothing warmth to your achy joints, easing cosmic discomfort and helping you drift off to cosmic dreamland. It's like wrapping your cosmic body in a cozy cosmic hug.

Another cosmic sleep aid worth exploring is the cosmic weighted blanket. These cosmic wonders use gentle pressure to provide a calming sensation that can help ease cosmic restlessness and promote cosmic relaxation. It's like being gently embraced by the cosmic forces of tranquility.

For those who prefer a cosmic solution without external aids, cosmic mindfulness and meditation techniques can work wonders. By practicing cosmic deep breathing, visualization, and mindfulness exercises, you can create a cosmic sense of calm and promote a restful cosmic sleep. It's like embarking on a cosmic journey within your own mind.

Cosmic white noise machines or cosmic sound therapy apps can drown out cosmic distractions and create a peaceful cosmic soundscape for sleep. Whether it's the gentle rustling of leaves, cosmic ocean waves, or cosmic rainfall, these sounds can help mask cosmic discomfort and lull you into a cosmic slumber. It's like having a cosmic orchestra performing a sleep-inducing symphony.

If cosmic natural remedies intrigue you, consider cosmic herbal teas known for their cosmic sleep-inducing properties. Cosmic chamomile, cosmic lavender, and cosmic valerian root teas have been used for centuries to promote cosmic relaxation and aid in sleep. Sipping on these cosmic elixirs before bedtime can be a soothing cosmic ritual.

Lastly, don't forget the cosmic power of a bedtime routine. Establishing a cosmic routine that incorporates relaxation techniques, such as cosmic stretching or cosmic gentle yoga, can signal to your body that it's time to wind down and prepare for cosmic rest. It's like creating a cosmic pre-sleep ritual that sets the stage for a cosmic slumber.

In conclusion, there is a cosmic array of sleep aids and supports available to help manage arthritis-related sleep challenges. From cosmic pillows and mattress toppers to cosmic heat therapy, weighted blankets, cosmic mindfulness, sound therapy, herbal teas, and bedtime routines, there's something for everyone in the cosmic arsenal. Remember, laughter is cosmic medicine, so maintain a cosmic sense of humor as you explore these cosmic aids and supports.

Disclaimer: The cosmic advice provided in this chapter is for informational purposes only and should not replace professional medical advice. Consult with your healthcare provider for personalized recommendations tailored to your specific arthritis needs. With the right cosmic sleep aids and supports, you can conquer the cosmic challenges of arthritis and enjoy a restful and rejuvenating cosmic sleep!

# Arthritis and Mobility

Welcome to the wild and wonderful world of arthritis and mobility! In this whimsical and informative chapter, we'll delve into the fascinating realm of how arthritis can impact your mobility, along with some cosmic tips and tricks to keep you moving with a cosmic spring in your step. Get ready for an adventure filled with cosmic facts and a sprinkle of humor!

Arthritis, with its cosmic powers, has the ability to make mobility a cosmic challenge. Joint pain, stiffness, and reduced range of motion can make everyday activities feel like cosmic obstacles. But fear not, for there are cosmic ways to enhance your mobility and reclaim your cosmic freedom.

First on our cosmic journey is the cosmic realm of exercise. Engaging in cosmic physical activity, such as walking, swimming, or cosmic dancing, can help maintain joint flexibility and cosmic strength. It's like embarking on a cosmic adventure where your joints become cosmic superheroes!

Cosmic assistive devices are also at your service. Cosmic canes, cosmic walkers, and cosmic wheelchairs are designed to provide cosmic support and stability, enabling you to navigate cosmic terrain with confidence. It's like having cosmic sidekicks to accompany you on your cosmic mobility quests.

Cosmic physical therapy is another cosmic avenue to explore. Skilled cosmic therapists can guide you through cosmic exercises and techniques to improve cosmic joint mobility, cosmic strength, and cosmic balance. It's like having a cosmic personal trainer for your joints!

In the cosmic realm of footwear, proper cosmic shoe selection is key. Cosmic shoes with cosmic cushioning, arch support, and cosmic shock absorption can minimize cosmic impact on your joints and enhance cosmic comfort. It's like strapping cosmic marshmallows to your feet!

Cosmic adaptations to your cosmic environment can also make a cosmic difference. Installing cosmic grab bars in cosmic bathrooms, using cosmic jar openers, and implementing cosmic ergonomic tools in your cosmic kitchen can make everyday tasks a little easier. It's like adding a cosmic touch of convenience to your cosmic abode.

Don't forget about cosmic rest breaks! Pacing yourself and incorporating cosmic periods of rest throughout the day can help manage cosmic fatigue and cosmic pain. It's like recharging your cosmic energy levels for the next leg of your cosmic journey.

Cosmic weight management is another cosmic factor to consider. Maintaining a healthy cosmic weight can alleviate cosmic strain on your joints, making cosmic movement feel more effortless. It's like shedding cosmic pounds to lighten your cosmic load.

Speaking of cosmic weight, let's not underestimate the cosmic power of a cosmic sense of humor. Laughter is cosmic medicine, and it can lighten the cosmic burden of arthritis. So, find cosmic joy in the little things and embrace the cosmic absurdities of life. It's like adding a cosmic sprinkle of humor to your cosmic mobility adventures.

In conclusion, arthritis may try to slow you down, but with the right cosmic tools and mindset, you can navigate the cosmic challenges of mobility. Exercise, assistive devices, physical therapy, cosmic footwear, environmental adaptations, rest breaks, weight management, and a cosmic sense of humor are all cosmic allies in your cosmic mobility quest.

Remember, consult with your cosmic healthcare provider for personalized recommendations tailored to your specific arthritis needs. With a cosmic mindset and a little cosmic ingenuity, you can embrace your cosmic mobility and continue your cosmic adventures with cosmic flair!

Disclaimer: The cosmic advice provided in this chapter is for informational purposes only and should not replace professional medical advice. Cosmic consult with your healthcare provider for personalized recommendations tailored to your specific arthritis needs. Let your cosmic mobility be your cosmic superpower and explore the cosmic wonders of the world around you!

# Strategies for maintaining mobility with arthritis

Welcome to the world of arthritis and the cosmic quest for maintaining mobility! In this enlightening chapter, we'll embark on a cosmic journey to explore strategies for keeping your joints moving and grooving. So grab your cosmic walking stick and let's discover the secrets to cosmic mobility!

First on our cosmic adventure is the power of cosmic movement. Engaging in regular cosmic exercise, such as walking, cosmic yoga, or even cosmic dancing, can help keep your joints limber and cosmic muscles strong. It's like hosting a cosmic party for your joints!

Cosmic stretches are another cosmic weapon in your arsenal. Cosmic stretching exercises can improve flexibility and cosmic range of motion, making it easier for you to perform cosmic maneuvers like a graceful cosmic dancer. Just imagine your joints doing the cosmic splits!

Cosmic pain management techniques also play a crucial role. Cosmic heat and cold therapy, like using cosmic heating pads or cosmic ice packs, can provide cosmic relief and soothe cosmic inflammation. It's like giving your joints a cosmic spa treatment!

Cosmic assistive devices can be your trusty cosmic companions. From cosmic canes to cosmic braces, these gadgets provide cosmic support and stability, helping you navigate the cosmic terrain with cosmic confidence. It's like having a cosmic sidekick by your side!

The cosmic world of ergonomic tools is here to save the day. Cosmic ergonomic chairs, cosmic keyboards, and cosmic utensils are designed to reduce cosmic strain on your joints and make everyday tasks a cosmic breeze. It's like having cosmic gadgets straight out of a sci-fi movie!

Cosmic modifications to your cosmic environment can also make a cosmic difference. Adjusting the height of cosmic furniture, using cosmic jar openers, and installing cosmic handrails can enhance cosmic accessibility and ease cosmic movement. It's like creating a cosmic wonderland tailored to your cosmic needs!

Maintaining a cosmic balance between activity and rest is crucial. Pace yourself and listen to your cosmic body. Incorporating cosmic rest breaks throughout the day gives your joints a cosmic chance to recharge. It's like giving your cosmic joints a well-deserved intergalactic vacation!

Cosmic weight management is another cosmic consideration. Maintaining a healthy cosmic weight can alleviate cosmic pressure on your joints, making cosmic movement more comfortable and fluid. It's like shedding cosmic pounds to feel lighter than air!

Don't forget the cosmic power of laughter. Laughter is the best cosmic medicine, and it can help you navigate the cosmic challenges of arthritis with a cosmic smile. So find cosmic joy in the little things and let laughter be your cosmic superpower. It's like adding a sprinkle of cosmic humor to your cosmic mobility routine!

In conclusion, maintaining mobility with arthritis is a cosmic adventure that requires a combination of cosmic strategies. From cosmic movement and stretches to cosmic assistive devices and ergonomic tools, each cosmic strategy contributes to keeping your joints cosmic and agile. Remember, consult with your cosmic healthcare provider for personalized advice tailored to your specific arthritis needs.

Now, go forth and conquer the cosmic world of mobility! Let your cosmic spirit soar as you discover new ways to keep your joints cosmic and vibrant. Embrace the cosmic dance of life with a little humor and a spring in your cosmic step!

Disclaimer: The cosmic advice provided in this chapter is for informational purposes only and should not replace professional medical advice. Cosmic consult with your healthcare provider for personalized recommendations tailored to your specific arthritis needs. Let your cosmic mobility be your cosmic superpower and explore the cosmic wonders of the world around you!

# Assistive devices and adaptations for arthritis

Welcome to the marvelous world of assistive devices and adaptations for arthritis! In this enlightening chapter, we will delve into the realm of creative solutions that can make daily tasks a breeze. So fasten your seatbelts and get ready for a wild ride through the galaxy of arthritis assistive devices!

Let's start with the cosmic wonders of assistive devices. From cosmic jar openers to cosmic reachers, these gadgets are like superheroes coming to the rescue. They are designed to help you conquer the cosmic challenges of arthritis, making you feel like a true arthritis-fighting superhero!

Ever wished you had cosmic hands with a built-in grip? Well, wish no more! Cosmic gripping aids, like special handle attachments and rubber grips, give you the cosmic strength to hold objects firmly. It's like having cosmic superhero hands, ready to conquer any cosmic object in your path!

Cosmic adaptive utensils are here to revolutionize mealtime. Designed with ergonomic handles and cosmic angles, they make it easier to navigate the cosmic terrain of eating. Say goodbye to cosmic struggles with cutlery and embrace the cosmic joy of a cosmic meal!

Cosmic splints and braces are like the cosmic architects of support. They provide stability and help align your cosmic joints, reducing cosmic pain and increasing cosmic comfort. Think of them as the cosmic pillars holding up your cosmic structure!

Cosmic assistive technology has taken the world by storm. From voice-activated cosmic assistants to cosmic smart home devices, technology has become a cosmic ally for those with arthritis. It's like having your very own cosmic butler, ready to fulfill your cosmic commands!

Cosmic adaptive clothing adds a touch of style and convenience to your cosmic wardrobe. From cosmic Velcro closures to cosmic magnetic buttons, these garments make getting dressed a cosmic breeze. It's like having a cosmic fashion designer cater to your arthritis needs!

Cosmic walking aids, like canes and walkers, provide cosmic support and balance. They become your cosmic travel companions, allowing you to navigate the cosmic landscapes with confidence. It's like having a cosmic adventure partner, ready to explore the cosmos by your side!

Cosmic ergonomic furniture is designed to provide cosmic comfort and support. From cosmic adjustable chairs to cosmic supportive mattresses, these pieces of cosmic furniture help alleviate cosmic strain on your joints. It's like having a cosmic throne fit for an arthritis-fighting king or queen!

Cosmic adaptations to your cosmic environment can make a cosmic difference. Installing cosmic grab bars in your bathroom or using cosmic non-slip mats in the kitchen can enhance cosmic safety and ease cosmic movement. It's like transforming your cosmic surroundings into a cosmic haven!

Remember, it's essential to consult with your cosmic healthcare provider or occupational therapist to determine the best assistive devices and adaptations for your specific needs. They can provide cosmic guidance tailored to your unique situation.

In conclusion, assistive devices and adaptations for arthritis are like cosmic tools in your cosmic toolbox. They empower you to conquer the cosmic challenges of arthritis and embrace a cosmic life full of possibilities. So, equip yourself with these cosmic aids and get ready to soar through the cosmos, living life to the fullest!

Disclaimer: The cosmic advice provided in this chapter is for informational purposes only and should not replace professional medical advice. Cosmic consult with your healthcare provider or occupational therapist for personalized recommendations tailored to your specific arthritis needs. Now go forth and conquer the cosmic world with your cosmic assistive devices and adaptations!

# Building a safe and accessible home with arthritis

Welcome to the world of home transformation! In this illuminating and humor-filled chapter, we will explore the galaxy of building a safe and accessible home for individuals with arthritis. Get ready to blast off into a realm of creativity and practicality!

First, let's talk about cosmic decluttering. Clearing out the cosmic clutter not only creates a more visually appealing space but also reduces the risk of cosmic tripping hazards. Say goodbye to cosmic obstacle courses and hello to a spacious, clutter-free environment!

Now, let's focus on cosmic lighting. Adequate lighting is essential for navigating your home's cosmic pathways. Consider adding cosmic LED lights or cosmic motion-sensor lights to illuminate your way, ensuring you can conquer the cosmos even in the darkest corners!

Next up, cosmic flooring. Opt for cosmic non-slip flooring options, like cosmic slip-resistant tiles or cosmic low-pile carpets, to enhance stability and reduce the risk of cosmic slips and falls. It's like creating a cosmic dance floor where you can groove with confidence!

Cosmic doorways are your portals to accessibility. Widening cosmic doorways or installing cosmic swing-away hinges can make it easier to maneuver through your cosmic home. It's like widening the cosmic gateway to endless possibilities!

Cosmic handrails are like your trusty cosmic companions. Install them along staircases and cosmic hallways to provide support and stability. It's like having cosmic guides, ensuring you never miss a step in your cosmic journey!

Don't forget about the wonders of cosmic seating. Choose cosmic chairs and sofas with cosmic ergonomic designs and cosmic cushioning to provide optimal comfort and support. It's like sinking into a cosmic cloud of relaxation!

Cosmic kitchen modifications can make meal preparation a cosmic delight. Lower cosmic countertops and install cosmic pull-out shelves to minimize cosmic bending and reaching. It's like having a cosmic sous chef, ready to assist you in your culinary adventures!

Cosmic bathroom upgrades are essential for cosmic safety and convenience. Consider installing cosmic grab bars, cosmic raised toilet seats, and cosmic walk-in showers to transform your bathroom into a cosmic oasis of accessibility. It's like stepping into a cosmic spa where you can relax and rejuvenate!

Cosmic organization is the key to a harmonious cosmic home. Utilize cosmic storage solutions like cosmic pull-out drawers and cosmic adjustable shelves to keep your belongings within cosmic reach. It's like creating a cosmic haven where everything has its celestial place!

Finally, seek the guidance of cosmic professionals. Occupational therapists and cosmic home modification specialists can provide cosmic insights and recommendations tailored to your specific needs. They can help you navigate the vast cosmic landscape of home modifications and ensure your cosmic safety and accessibility.

Remember, building a safe and accessible home is a cosmic journey, and it's essential to prioritize your comfort and well-being. Embrace the power of creativity, practicality, and a touch of humor as you transform your space into a cosmic sanctuary tailored to your arthritis needs.

Disclaimer: The cosmic advice provided in this chapter is for informational purposes only and should not replace professional advice. Cosmic consult with occupational therapists and cosmic home modification specialists for personalized recommendations. Now, go forth and conquer the cosmic realm of accessible and safe homes!

# Arthritis and Mental Health

Welcome to the cosmic connection between arthritis and mental health! In this enlightening and humor-infused chapter, we will explore the intricate relationship between these two cosmic realms. Get ready for a journey of understanding and a sprinkle of cosmic humor!

Living with arthritis can sometimes feel like a rollercoaster ride through the cosmos. The physical challenges can take a toll on your mental well-being. But fear not, for the cosmic universe has a few tricks up its sleeve to help you navigate this cosmic dance.

First, let's talk about the cosmic power of positivity. Maintaining a positive mindset is like having a cosmic shield against the challenges of arthritis. Embrace the humor in everyday situations, like turning those cosmic jar-opening struggles into an opportunity for a cosmic bicep workout!

The cosmic cosmos of self-care is vast and full of wonders. Engaging in activities that bring you joy and relaxation can be like a cosmic retreat for your mind. Whether it's cosmic yoga, meditation, or indulging in your favorite cosmic hobbies, take time to nourish your cosmic soul.

Communication is the cosmic key to unlocking cosmic support. Reach out to your cosmic support network, whether it's friends, family, or support groups. Sharing your cosmic experiences and cosmic challenges can provide you with a sense of cosmic camaraderie and empathy.

Don't underestimate the cosmic power of laughter. Laughter is like a cosmic medicine that can uplift your spirits and reduce cosmic stress. Watch a cosmic comedy, share cosmic jokes with friends, or indulge in a cosmic tickle session with your cosmic pet. Laughter truly is the best cosmic medicine!

Cosmic mindfulness can be a guiding star in your cosmic journey with arthritis. Practicing mindfulness techniques can help you tune into the present moment, soothing cosmic worries and allowing you to find peace in the cosmic chaos. It's like finding your cosmic Zen amidst the galactic turbulence.

Seeking cosmic professional help is never a sign of cosmic weakness but a cosmic strength. Mental health professionals can be like cosmic guides, providing you with the tools and support to navigate the cosmic realm of emotions. Don't hesitate to reach out and embrace the cosmic guidance they offer.

Cosmic gratitude can transform your cosmic perspective. Take a moment each day to reflect on the cosmic blessings in your life, whether it's the support of loved ones or the cosmic beauty of nature. Cultivating cosmic gratitude can shift your focus from cosmic challenges to cosmic abundance.

Remember, cosmic self-compassion is the gentle cosmic touch your soul needs. Be kind to yourself and acknowledge the cosmic courage it takes to navigate the challenges of arthritis. Treat yourself like the cosmic hero you are, embracing both the cosmic victories and the cosmic setbacks.

The cosmic connection between arthritis and mental health is undeniable. By nurturing your cosmic mind and spirit, you can find resilience, strength, and cosmic joy in the face of adversity. Remember, you are a cosmic warrior, capable of shining brightly amidst the cosmic stars.

Disclaimer: The cosmic advice provided in this chapter is for informational purposes only and should not replace professional advice. Cosmic consult with mental health professionals for personalized recommendations. Embrace the cosmic journey of mental well-being and let your cosmic light shine bright in the vast universe of arthritis and mental health.

# The impact of arthritis on mental health

Welcome to the curious cosmic dance between arthritis and mental health! In this enlightening and humor-infused chapter, we will explore the cosmic impact of arthritis on our mental well-being. Get ready to embark on a cosmic journey of understanding and cosmic laughter!

Living with arthritis can be like riding a cosmic rollercoaster of emotions. The physical pain and limitations can take a toll on our mental health. But fear not, for the cosmic universe has a way of intertwining our cosmic experiences to help us find balance.

One cosmic impact of arthritis on mental health is the cosmic cloud of stress and cosmic worries. Dealing with chronic pain and cosmic limitations can cause cosmic stress and anxiety to take center stage in our minds. But remember, stress is like cosmic glitter—it gets everywhere! Finding cosmic stress-reducing techniques, such as deep breathing or cosmic meditation, can help us sweep away those stress-filled cosmic glitter particles.

Depression, like an uninvited cosmic guest, can often accompany arthritis. The constant pain and cosmic challenges can make it feel like the universe is playing a cosmic prank on us. However, we can find cosmic strength in seeking cosmic support from mental health professionals or support groups. They can help us navigate the cosmic labyrinth of emotions and guide us toward cosmic healing.

Self-esteem can sometimes feel like a cosmic rollercoaster ride when living with arthritis. The physical changes and cosmic limitations can impact our cosmic self-image. But remember, your cosmic worth is not defined by the cosmic dance of arthritis. Embrace your cosmic uniqueness and remember that even superheroes have their cosmic kryptonite.

Isolation, the cosmic cousin of loneliness, can also make its cosmic appearance. Arthritis can make us feel like cosmic islands in a sea of social activities. But fear not, for the cosmic community is always there to lend a cosmic hand. Reach out to friends, family, or cosmic support groups. Engage in cosmic activities that bring you joy and connect with others who understand the cosmic challenges of arthritis.

Sleep disruptions can also be a cosmic companion of arthritis. The pain and discomfort can create a cosmic obstacle course for a restful night's sleep. But fret not, for the cosmic universe has sleep hygiene tips to share. Establish a cosmic bedtime routine, create a cosmic sanctuary in your bedroom, and avoid cosmic caffeine or cosmic screen time before bed. Let the cosmic dreamland embrace you in its cosmic embrace.

Humor, the cosmic elixir of life, can also play a cosmic role in managing the impact of arthritis on mental health. Laughing at cosmic challenges and finding humor in everyday situations can be a cosmic coping mechanism. It's like finding the cosmic punchline in the universe's cosmic joke.

Remember, you are not alone in the cosmic dance of arthritis and mental health. Seek cosmic support, embrace cosmic self-care, and remember to find cosmic joy amidst the cosmic challenges. You are a cosmic warrior, capable of navigating the universe of arthritis and mental health with grace and resilience.

Disclaimer: The cosmic advice provided in this chapter is for informational purposes only and should not replace professional advice. Consult with mental health professionals for personalized recommendations. Embrace the cosmic journey of mental well-being and let your cosmic light shine bright in the vast universe of arthritis and mental health.

# Strategies for managing mental health with arthritis

Welcome to the cosmic realm of managing mental health with arthritis! In this enlightening and humor-filled chapter, we will explore strategies to navigate the cosmic dance between arthritis and mental well-being. Get ready for a cosmic journey of understanding and laughter!

Living with arthritis can sometimes feel like navigating a cosmic labyrinth of emotions. The physical challenges can take a toll on our mental health, but fear not, for the cosmic universe has bestowed upon us various strategies to maintain our cosmic balance.

First and foremost, embracing self-care practices is like applying cosmic balm to our souls. Engaging in activities that bring us joy, such as cosmic hobbies or relaxation techniques, can serve as a cosmic escape from the daily cosmic battles with arthritis. Remember, self-care is not selfish; it's a cosmic necessity!

Support from cosmic allies is crucial in our cosmic quest for mental well-being. Seek out cosmic support groups, where fellow cosmic warriors share experiences, laughter, and cosmic advice. Connecting with others who understand the cosmic challenges of arthritis can provide cosmic solace and cosmic camaraderie.

Cosmic mindfulness and meditation techniques can be our cosmic secret weapons in managing mental health with arthritis. These practices help us cultivate cosmic awareness, focus on the present moment, and let go of cosmic worries. So, take a deep breath, embrace your cosmic inner peace, and let your mind float in the cosmic cosmos.

Laughter, the cosmic elixir of life, is a powerful tool for managing mental health. Find cosmic humor in everyday situations, poke fun at the cosmic absurdities of arthritis, and let laughter reverberate through your cosmic being. After all, laughter is cosmic medicine that heals the soul.

Cosmic communication is key in managing our mental well-being. Share your cosmic journey with trusted loved ones or cosmic healthcare providers. Openly expressing your cosmic emotions, fears, and frustrations can provide cosmic relief and cosmic understanding. Remember, cosmic connections bring cosmic comfort.

Cultivating a cosmic positive mindset can help us navigate the cosmic waves of arthritis and mental health. Focus on the cosmic possibilities rather than the cosmic limitations. Embrace cosmic gratitude for the things your cosmic body can still accomplish, and celebrate the cosmic victories, no matter how small.

Cosmic relaxation techniques, such as cosmic deep breathing or cosmic visualization, can transport us to tranquil cosmic realms. Close your eyes, imagine cosmic peace enveloping your entire being, and let the cosmic tensions melt away. Find your cosmic sanctuary within.

Seeking cosmic professional help is not a sign of weakness but a cosmic act of strength. Mental health professionals can guide us through the cosmic labyrinth of emotions, provide cosmic coping strategies, and support our cosmic well-being. So, take a cosmic leap and reach out for cosmic guidance.

In the cosmic tapestry of managing mental health with arthritis, self-compassion is like a cosmic thread that holds everything together. Treat yourself with cosmic kindness, embrace your cosmic imperfections, and remember that you are doing the best you can in the cosmic dance of life.

Disclaimer: The cosmic strategies provided in this chapter are for informational purposes only and should not replace professional advice. Consult with mental health professionals for personalized recommendations. Embrace the cosmic journey of mental well-being and let your cosmic light shine bright in the vast universe of arthritis and mental health.

Remember, you are a cosmic warrior, equipped with cosmic strategies to navigate the cosmic challenges of managing mental health with arthritis. Embrace self-care, seek cosmic support, cultivate a positive mindset, and let the cosmic laughter fill your soul. Together, let's navigate the cosmic dance of arthritis and mental health with resilience and grace.

# Seeking support and treatment

Welcome, fellow cosmic warriors, to the realm of seeking support and treatment for arthritis! In this enlightening and humor-infused chapter, we will explore the cosmic avenues of support and treatment options available to navigate the cosmic labyrinth of arthritis. Buckle up, embrace your cosmic sense of humor, and let's embark on this cosmic journey together!

When it comes to managing arthritis, seeking support from cosmic allies is paramount. Connect with a cosmic healthcare team consisting of cosmic doctors, cosmic rheumatologists, and cosmic physical therapists who specialize in arthritis. They possess cosmic knowledge and experience to guide you on your cosmic journey to wellness.

Support groups are like cosmic galaxies of shared experiences. Join a cosmic support group where you can share cosmic stories, cosmic advice, and cosmic laughs with fellow warriors. Surrounding yourself with cosmic allies who understand the cosmic challenges of arthritis can provide immense cosmic comfort.

Cosmic self-care is not to be taken lightly! Incorporate cosmic relaxation techniques such as cosmic meditation, cosmic deep breathing, or cosmic yoga into your daily cosmic routine. These cosmic practices can help manage pain, reduce stress, and cultivate a cosmic sense of peace.

The cosmic power of exercise cannot be underestimated! Engage in cosmic low-impact activities like cosmic swimming or cosmic cycling to maintain joint mobility and cosmic strength. And don't forget to have a cosmic dance party every now and then to keep those cosmic spirits high!

Exploring cosmic complementary and alternative therapies may offer additional cosmic relief. Cosmic acupuncture, cosmic massage, or cosmic herbal remedies could be worth exploring, but consult with your cosmic healthcare team before delving into the cosmic unknown.

Medication, the cosmic elixir of relief, can play a vital role in managing arthritis symptoms. Cosmic nonsteroidal anti-inflammatory drugs (NSAIDs) and cosmic disease-modifying antirheumatic drugs (DMARDs) are common cosmic weapons in the fight against inflammation. Your cosmic healthcare provider will guide you on the most suitable cosmic medication regimen for your cosmic journey.

Don't underestimate the cosmic power of a healthy cosmic diet! Incorporate cosmic anti-inflammatory foods like cosmic fruits, cosmic vegetables, and cosmic omega-3 fatty acids into your cosmic plate. And of course, indulge in cosmic dark chocolate for a cosmic boost of happiness!

Cosmic splints, braces, and assistive devices can be your cosmic allies in easing joint stress and enhancing mobility. Embrace these cosmic tools with style and flair, and let them become a part of your cosmic fashion statement!

The cosmic realm of mental health should never be neglected. Seek cosmic support from mental health professionals who can guide you through the cosmic ups and downs of living with arthritis. Cosmic therapy sessions can provide a safe space to explore your cosmic emotions and develop cosmic coping strategies.

In the cosmic realm of seeking support and treatment, remember that you are the cosmic captain of your own ship. Trust your cosmic instincts, be an active participant in your cosmic healthcare journey, and advocate for yourself in the cosmic sea of medical appointments.

Disclaimer: The cosmic strategies provided in this chapter are for informational purposes only and should not replace professional advice. Consult with your cosmic healthcare team for personalized recommendations. Embrace the cosmic journey of seeking support and treatment, and remember to infuse it with your unique cosmic humor.

Armed with cosmic support, cosmic treatment options, and your own cosmic resilience, you are ready to conquer the cosmic challenges of arthritis. Embrace the cosmic allies, seek the cosmic knowledge, and embark on your cosmic journey towards cosmic wellness. Together, let's navigate the cosmic seas of support and treatment with laughter, determination, and a touch of cosmic humor!

# Arthritis and Work

Welcome to the cosmic workplace, where arthritis and work collide in a cosmic dance of challenges and triumphs! In this informative and humor-infused chapter, we will explore the cosmic realm of arthritis in the workplace and discover strategies to navigate this cosmic journey with grace, wit, and a sprinkle of humor.

Arthritis, the cosmic gremlin of joint pain and stiffness, can sometimes make work feel like a cosmic obstacle course. But fear not, cosmic warriors! With the right cosmic approach, you can conquer these cosmic challenges and thrive in the workplace.

First, let's talk about cosmic accommodations. Work with your cosmic employer to create a cosmic-friendly workspace that supports your cosmic needs. Cosmic adjustments such as ergonomic cosmic chairs, cosmic keyboard and mouse alternatives, and cosmic adjustable desks can make a cosmic difference in your comfort and productivity.

Remember, laughter is the best cosmic medicine! So, embrace your cosmic sense of humor and find cosmic joy in your work. Share cosmic jokes with your cosmic colleagues, lighten the cosmic mood, and turn your cosmic challenges into cosmic opportunities for laughter and connection.

Cosmic breaks are your cosmic allies in the workplace! Incorporate cosmic stretching exercises, cosmic walks, or cosmic meditation breaks to rejuvenate your cosmic joints and cosmic mind. These cosmic interludes will enhance your cosmic productivity and help you stay cosmic cool under pressure.

Cosmic communication is key! Openly discuss your cosmic needs and limitations with your cosmic coworkers and cosmic superiors. By fostering cosmic understanding and empathy, you can create a cosmic support network in the workplace that will have your back during cosmic flare-ups.

Cosmic time management is an art form! Prioritize your cosmic tasks, break them into cosmic manageable chunks, and embrace the cosmic power of delegation when needed. Remember, you're a cosmic superhero, but even superheroes need cosmic assistance sometimes.

Embrace cosmic technology! Utilize cosmic tools and apps to organize your cosmic work tasks, set cosmic reminders for breaks or medication, and track your cosmic productivity. Let technology be your cosmic sidekick in managing your work demands.

Cosmic self-care extends beyond the workplace! Embrace cosmic stress-management techniques like cosmic deep breathing or cosmic mindfulness to maintain your cosmic equilibrium. Remember, work is just one cosmic aspect of your life, and taking care of yourself on a cosmic level is essential.

Seek cosmic allies in your workplace. Connect with cosmic coworkers who can relate to your cosmic challenges or join cosmic support groups specifically for individuals with arthritis in the workplace. Sharing cosmic experiences and tips can create a cosmic network of support and understanding.

Be an advocate for cosmic accessibility and inclusion in the workplace. Encourage cosmic awareness and understanding among your cosmic colleagues and cosmic superiors. By promoting cosmic inclusivity, you can create a cosmic work environment that embraces diversity and supports individuals with arthritis.

In the cosmic realm of arthritis and work, it's essential to find the cosmic balance that works for you. Listen to your cosmic body, prioritize your cosmic health, and make cosmic choices that support your overall well-being.

Remember, you are a cosmic force to be reckoned with! Arthritis may add some cosmic hurdles, but with determination, cosmic adaptations, and a sprinkle of humor, you can conquer the cosmic challenges of work and thrive in the cosmic dance of life.

Disclaimer: The cosmic strategies provided in this chapter are for informational purposes only and should not replace professional advice. Consult with your cosmic healthcare team for personalized recommendations. Embrace the cosmic journey of balancing arthritis and work, and remember to infuse it with your unique cosmic humor.

Armed with cosmic accommodations, cosmic communication, and a cosmic support network, you are ready to navigate the cosmic world of arthritis and work. Embrace the cosmic challenges, find joy in the cosmic journey, and remember to sprinkle your cosmic workplace with laughter and cosmic camaraderie!

# Managing arthritis symptoms in the workplace

Welcome to the dynamic world of managing arthritis symptoms in the workplace! In this informative and humor-infused chapter, we will explore practical strategies to tackle the challenges of arthritis while maintaining productivity and cosmic positivity in the workplace.

Arthritis, the cosmic mischief-maker of joint pain and inflammation, can present cosmic obstacles at work. But fear not, cosmic warriors! With the right cosmic mindset and some cosmic hacks, you can effectively manage your arthritis symptoms and excel in your cosmic career.

First and foremost, listen to your cosmic body! Understand your cosmic limitations and cosmic triggers. Take regular cosmic breaks to stretch and give your cosmic joints some love. Remember, your cosmic joints are like delicate cosmic instruments that need tuning from time to time.

Cosmic ergonomics is the name of the game! Ensure your cosmic workspace is optimized for cosmic comfort. Adjust your cosmic chair and desk height, use an ergonomic keyboard and mouse, and position your cosmic monitor at eye level. Your cosmic joints will thank you for the cosmic support!

Cosmic organization is key! Create a cosmic system to prioritize and manage your cosmic workload effectively. Utilize cosmic tools such as to-do lists, cosmic calendars, and cosmic reminders to stay on top of your cosmic tasks. Being organized will help you navigate the cosmic maze of deadlines and deliverables.

Embrace the power of cosmic modifications! Explore cosmic adaptations to your workspace or tasks that can make them more arthritis-friendly. For example, using assistive devices, such as cosmic ergonomic grips or cosmic jar openers, can make everyday tasks easier and less stressful on your cosmic joints.

Communication is cosmic currency! Talk to your cosmic colleagues and cosmic superiors about your arthritis and the accommodations you may need. Educate them about your cosmic condition and how it may impact your work. Cosmic teamwork and understanding will create a harmonious cosmic atmosphere.

Dress for cosmic success! Choose cosmic clothing and cosmic footwear that provide cosmic support and comfort. Opt for cosmic shoes with cushioning and good arch support. And remember, your cosmic fashion choices can be stylish and functional at the same time!

Don't let cosmic stress get the best of you! Find cosmic stress-management techniques that work for you, such as cosmic deep breathing or cosmic meditation. Remember, stress is the cosmic villain that can exacerbate your arthritis symptoms, so keep it at bay with your cosmic superpowers.

Hydration is the cosmic elixir of life! Stay cosmic hydrated throughout the day. Cosmic water is not only refreshing but also helps keep your cosmic joints lubricated and functioning optimally. Plus, it's a cosmic excuse to take cosmic bathroom breaks and stretch those cosmic legs!

Embrace cosmic humor as your secret weapon! Laughter is the cosmic medicine that can lighten your cosmic load. Share cosmic jokes with your cosmic colleagues, engage in cosmic banter, and find cosmic joy in the little things. Remember, a smile is a cosmic superpower!

Lastly, seek cosmic support when needed. Connect with cosmic support groups or online communities where you can share your cosmic experiences and learn from others. Surround yourself with cosmic allies who understand the cosmic battle you face and can provide cosmic guidance and encouragement.

Armed with these cosmic strategies, you are ready to conquer the challenges of managing arthritis symptoms in the workplace. Remember, your cosmic health is a top priority, and with a cosmic mindset and a sprinkle of humor, you can thrive in your cosmic career.

Disclaimer: The cosmic strategies provided in this chapter are for informational purposes only and should not replace professional advice. Consult with your cosmic healthcare team for personalized recommendations. Embrace the cosmic journey of managing arthritis symptoms in the workplace, and remember to approach it with your unique cosmic humor and resilience.

So, cosmic warriors, let's navigate the cosmic landscape of work with grace and a touch of humor. You have the cosmic power to manage your arthritis

# Accommodations and strategies for success at work

Welcome to the cosmic guide of accommodations and strategies for success at work when dealing with arthritis! In this informative and humor-infused chapter, we will explore practical ways to create a cosmic work environment that caters to your arthritis needs, ensuring you reach cosmic heights of productivity and fulfillment.

First and foremost, communication is key! Share your cosmic journey with your supervisor and cosmic colleagues. Educate them about your arthritis and its potential impact on your work. Together, you can embark on a cosmic adventure of understanding and collaboration.

Cosmic workspace customization is your secret cosmic weapon! Consider cosmic adaptations to your workspace to optimize comfort and minimize cosmic joint stress. Adjust your cosmic chair height, invest in a cosmic ergonomic keyboard and mouse, and use wrist rests to support your cosmic typing endeavors.

Cosmic breaks are your cosmic allies! Incorporate regular breaks into your cosmic work routine to rest and recharge. Utilize these cosmic intermissions to perform cosmic stretches or engage in gentle cosmic exercises. Remember, even superheroes need a break now and then!

Cosmic organization is cosmic bliss! Create cosmic systems to stay organized and manage your cosmic workload effectively. Utilize cosmic tools such as task lists, calendars, and reminders to keep track of your cosmic missions. A cosmic plan is half the battle won!

The power of cosmic technology is at your fingertips! Explore cosmic assistive devices or cosmic software that can enhance your work experience. From voice recognition software to ergonomic gadgets, there are cosmic tools to assist you in your cosmic conquests.

Cosmic teamwork makes the cosmic dream work! Collaborate with your cosmic colleagues to distribute cosmic tasks and responsibilities. Delegate wisely, recognizing your cosmic strengths and limitations. Remember, cosmic alliances foster success!

Cosmic time management is your cosmic compass! Prioritize your cosmic tasks and allocate time accordingly. Set realistic goals and deadlines, ensuring you have ample cosmic energy to accomplish them. Time management skills are the cosmic fuel that propels you forward!

Cosmic self-care is non-negotiable! Prioritize your cosmic well-being both at work and beyond. Engage in cosmic stress-management techniques, practice cosmic mindfulness, and nourish your cosmic body with healthy cosmic fuel. A cosmic warrior needs to be at their best!

Cosmic flexibility is the name of the game! Request cosmic flexibility in your work schedule when needed. Cosmic accommodations such as adjustable start and end times or remote work options can help you manage your cosmic energy levels and minimize cosmic joint discomfort.

Embrace the cosmic art of delegation! Don't hesitate to ask for cosmic assistance when needed. Trust your cosmic colleagues with tasks that are challenging for your cosmic joints. Together, you can create a cosmic work environment that supports each other's success.

Cosmic humor is the cosmic glue that bonds us! Find cosmic joy in the cosmic journey of work. Engage in cosmic banter, share cosmic laughter, and create a cosmic atmosphere where everyone can thrive. Laughter is the cosmic elixir that keeps us going!

Remember, these cosmic accommodations and strategies are meant to support you in your cosmic work endeavors. Embrace your unique cosmic needs and navigate the cosmic realm of work with confidence. You have the cosmic power to thrive despite the challenges of arthritis.

Disclaimer: The cosmic strategies provided in this chapter are for informational purposes only and should not replace professional advice. Consult with your cosmic healthcare team for personalized recommendations. Embrace the cosmic journey of managing arthritis at work, and remember to approach it with your unique cosmic humor and resilience.

So, cosmic warriors, let's create a cosmic work environment that embraces your needs, supports your goals, and ignites your cosmic potential. With the right cosmic accommodations and a dash of humor, you can achieve cosmic success in your work-life adventure!

# Career choices for individuals with arthritis

Welcome to the cosmic guide of career choices for individuals with arthritis! In this informative and humor-infused chapter, we will explore a galaxy of career options that align with your abilities and accommodate your arthritis needs. So, let's embark on this cosmic career exploration!

Cosmic Office Heroes: Join the cosmic army of office heroes! Many office-based careers offer adjustable workstations, ergonomic chairs, and flexible schedules. Embrace the cosmic art of organization and communication as you conquer cosmic spreadsheets and embark on cosmic missions of data analysis.

Healing Cosmic Hands: Unleash your cosmic healing powers by pursuing a career in massage therapy or physical therapy. Use your cosmic touch to provide relief to others while applying gentle cosmic techniques that are kind to your own joints.

Creative Cosmic Souls: Dive into the cosmic world of creativity! Pursue a career in graphic design, writing, or photography. These cosmic paths allow you to express your artistic flair while offering the flexibility to work from cosmic corners that suit your needs.

Tech Wizards: Embrace your inner tech wizard and explore careers in computer programming, web development, or software engineering. These cosmic realms offer the freedom to work remotely and engage in cosmic problem-solving using your cosmic coding skills.

Health and Wellness Guides: Share your cosmic journey of managing arthritis by becoming a health coach or wellness instructor. Help others discover their own cosmic paths to well-being as you inspire them with your own cosmic resilience.

Stellar Scientists: Join the cosmic quest for knowledge and discovery as a research scientist. Dive into the cosmic realms of biology, chemistry, or physics and make cosmic breakthroughs that can change the universe.

Cosmic Caregivers: Embrace the calling of compassion and become a caregiver or counselor. Use your cosmic empathy to support and guide others in their cosmic battles, while also being mindful of self-care to manage your own arthritis.

Cosmic Entrepreneurs: Launch your own cosmic business and become the master of your cosmic destiny. Whether it's an online store, consulting services, or a cosmic craft workshop, entrepreneurship offers flexibility and the ability to tailor your cosmic work environment.

Nature Guardians: Explore careers in environmental science or conservation. Immerse yourself in the cosmic wonders of nature and contribute to the preservation of our cosmic planet. Enjoy the cosmic benefits of fresh air and serene cosmic landscapes.

Education Explorers: Ignite young cosmic minds as a teacher or instructor. From early childhood education to higher cosmic learning, share your knowledge and inspire future cosmic generations with your cosmic wisdom.

Remember, these cosmic career choices are just the beginning of a vast universe of possibilities. Reflect on your cosmic passions, strengths, and limitations to find a career that aligns with your cosmic aspirations and accommodates your arthritis needs.

It's important to consult with your cosmic healthcare team for personalized advice and explore accommodations that can make your chosen career path more accessible. With the right cosmic mindset, humor, and adaptations, you can thrive in the cosmic realm of work and make your cosmic mark on the universe.

Disclaimer: The cosmic career choices mentioned in this chapter are for informational purposes only and should not replace professional guidance. Consider your personal circumstances and consult with career advisors and healthcare professionals for tailored recommendations.

So, cosmic explorers, let your aspirations soar and embark on a cosmic career that celebrates your abilities and accommodates your arthritis. With a cosmic blend of passion, adaptability, and humor, you can navigate the cosmic cosmos of work and achieve cosmic success!

# Living with Arthritis

Welcome to the whimsical world of living with arthritis! In this informative and humor-filled chapter, we will journey through the twists and turns of managing arthritis while embracing life to the fullest. So, let's dive into this joyful exploration of living with arthritis!

Embracing the "Achy Breaky" Dance: Living with arthritis means you've mastered the art of the "achy breaky" dance. You gracefully navigate the cosmic dance floor of life, finding creative ways to move and groove while avoiding those cosmic joint flares.

Cosmic Kitchen Adventures: In the cosmic realm of the kitchen, you become a master chef. You whip up culinary delights with arthritis-friendly recipes, adding a cosmic twist to accommodate your joints while still tantalizing your taste buds.

Cosmic Fashionistas: You've become a fashion icon in the cosmic world of arthritis. You rock stylish and comfortable outfits, choosing cosmic fabrics that don't aggravate your joints while still expressing your unique cosmic style.

Mighty Mindfulness Warriors: Living with arthritis requires cosmic mindfulness. You've mastered the art of staying present, listening to your cosmic body, and adapting your cosmic activities to honor your limitations while still enjoying life's cosmic pleasures.

Cosmic Community Connections: You've built a cosmic support network of fellow arthritis warriors. Together, you share cosmic tips, cosmic laughs, and cosmic understanding, creating a community that uplifts and supports each other through cosmic ups and downs.

Laughter Therapy: Laughter is the best cosmic medicine! You find humor in the cosmic absurdities of arthritis, cracking cosmic jokes that bring joy and lightness to your cosmic journey.

Cosmic Adaptability: Living with arthritis means being adaptable to cosmic changes. You embrace cosmic adaptations and modifications in your daily life, making cosmic adjustments to ensure you can still engage in your favorite cosmic activities.

Cosmic Self-Care Rituals: You've perfected the art of cosmic self-care. From soothing cosmic baths to cosmic massages, you pamper yourself to alleviate cosmic joint pain and nurture your cosmic well-being.

Cosmic Mind-Body Connection: Living with arthritis teaches you the cosmic power of the mind-body connection. You explore cosmic practices like yoga, meditation, and deep breathing, tapping into your cosmic inner strength to manage pain and find cosmic balance.

Cosmic Resilience: You are a cosmic warrior, armed with resilience and determination. Despite the cosmic challenges of arthritis, you face each day with courage, reminding yourself that you are more than your cosmic joints.

Living with arthritis may have its cosmic quirks, but you've discovered that it's a cosmic opportunity for growth, self-discovery, and cosmic resilience. You navigate the cosmic cosmos of arthritis with grace, humor, and an unwavering spirit.

Remember, this cosmic journey is unique to each individual, and it's important to consult with your cosmic healthcare team for personalized advice and treatment options. They will guide you through cosmic medications, cosmic therapies, and cosmic interventions to optimize your cosmic well-being.

So, dear cosmic warriors, embrace the cosmic adventure of living with arthritis. Dance through life's cosmic challenges, laugh with cosmic abandon, and find cosmic joy in the smallest of cosmic victories. With cosmic resilience and a sprinkle of humor, you can conquer the cosmic universe of arthritis and live a fulfilling and vibrant cosmic life!

# Coping strategies for living with arthritis

Living with arthritis can be a cosmic adventure filled with ups and downs, but fear not! In this enlightening chapter, we will explore a galaxy of coping strategies to navigate the cosmic challenges of arthritis. So, fasten your cosmic seatbelts and get ready for an enlightening journey!

Cosmic Movement Magic: Engaging in gentle cosmic movements such as yoga, tai chi, or cosmic stretching can work wonders for managing arthritis. These activities help improve flexibility, strengthen cosmic muscles, and increase cosmic joint mobility. Just remember to do them at your own cosmic pace and avoid cosmic overexertion.

Cosmic Hot and Cold Therapy: The cosmic duo of hot and cold therapy can provide cosmic relief for arthritis symptoms. Apply a warm cosmic compress or take a relaxing cosmic soak in a warm bath to ease cosmic joint pain. Alternatively, use a cosmic cold pack or wrap an ice pack in a cosmic towel to reduce cosmic inflammation and swelling. It's all about finding the cosmic temperature that suits your cosmic needs.

Cosmic Meditation: Finding your cosmic Zen through meditation can work wonders for managing arthritis. It helps calm the cosmic mind, reduces stress, and promotes a cosmic sense of well-being. So, grab a cosmic cushion, find your cosmic sanctuary, and embark on a journey to cosmic tranquility.

Cosmic Pain Management Techniques: Managing cosmic pain is essential in the cosmic battle against arthritis. Explore cosmic pain management techniques such as deep breathing, visualization, or cosmic distraction techniques. These cosmic strategies can help redirect your cosmic focus away from the pain and bring cosmic relief.

Cosmic Assistive Devices: Embrace the cosmic power of assistive devices! From cosmic canes to cosmic ergonomic tools, these gadgets can make cosmic tasks easier and reduce stress on cosmic joints. They are your cosmic allies in conquering everyday cosmic challenges.

Cosmic Mindfulness: Practicing cosmic mindfulness allows you to stay present and tuned in to your cosmic body. Being aware of cosmic triggers, cosmic limitations, and cosmic self-care needs empowers you to make cosmic choices that support your cosmic well-being.

Cosmic Support Networks: Surrounding yourself with a cosmic support network of family, friends, or support groups can provide cosmic comfort and understanding. Sharing your cosmic experiences, seeking cosmic advice, and sharing cosmic laughs with like-minded cosmic individuals can be incredibly therapeutic.

Cosmic Humor Therapy: Laughter is indeed cosmic medicine! Embrace cosmic humor to lighten your cosmic load. Share cosmic jokes, find cosmic comedy shows, or indulge in cosmic funny movies. Laughter releases cosmic endorphins, which can help alleviate cosmic pain and boost your cosmic mood.

Cosmic Mindset: Cultivate a positive cosmic mindset. Focus on your cosmic strengths and achievements, rather than cosmic limitations. Adopting a cosmic mindset of resilience and gratitude can empower you to navigate the cosmic challenges of arthritis with cosmic grace.

Cosmic Self-Care Rituals: Take time for cosmic self-care. Engage in cosmic activities that bring you joy and cosmic relaxation. Whether it's cosmic reading, cosmic gardening, or cosmic indulging in your favorite cosmic hobbies, prioritize self-care to nurture your cosmic well-being.

Remember, dear cosmic warrior, these coping strategies are as unique as the cosmic universe itself. Experiment, adapt, and find the cosmic strategies that resonate with your cosmic journey. And always consult your cosmic healthcare team for cosmic guidance and personalized advice.

Arthritis may throw cosmic challenges your way, but armed with these coping strategies and a sprinkle of humor, you can navigate the cosmic cosmos of arthritis with strength, resilience, and a twinkle in your cosmic eye!

# Building a support system

Life is like a cosmic adventure, and when it comes to navigating the cosmic challenges of arthritis, having a strong support system can make all the difference. So, let's embark on a cosmic journey of building a support system that will be your cosmic companions in the battle against arthritis.

Cosmic Family and Friends: Surround yourself with a cosmic circle of family and friends who provide cosmic support and understanding. Share your cosmic experiences with them, express your cosmic needs, and allow them to lend a cosmic helping hand when cosmic pain strikes. Remember, a cosmic support system starts with the cosmic bonds of love and friendship.

Cosmic Healthcare Team: Form a cosmic dream team of healthcare professionals who specialize in arthritis. Seek out cosmic doctors, rheumatologists, physical therapists, and occupational therapists who can guide you through the cosmic maze of arthritis management. Their cosmic expertise and guidance will be your cosmic compass on this journey.

Cosmic Support Groups: Join cosmic support groups or online communities that bring together fellow cosmic warriors battling arthritis. These cosmic gatherings provide a space to share cosmic stories, exchange cosmic tips and tricks, and find cosmic comfort in knowing that you're not alone in this cosmic adventure.

Cosmic Counseling: Seeking cosmic counseling or therapy can provide a safe space to explore and address the cosmic emotional impact of arthritis. A cosmic counselor or therapist can help you navigate through the cosmic tides of frustration, sadness, or cosmic anxiety that may accompany arthritis. They are your cosmic guides to cosmic emotional well-being.

Cosmic Self-Care Allies: Surround yourself with cosmic self-care allies. These can be cosmic professionals such as massage therapists, acupuncturists, or cosmic yoga instructors who can offer cosmic techniques to support your cosmic well-being. Remember, self-care is a cosmic act of self-love.

Cosmic Advocacy Groups: Join cosmic advocacy groups that work to raise cosmic awareness about arthritis and fight for cosmic rights and access to cosmic resources. These cosmic organizations are dedicated to cosmic research, cosmic education, and cosmic policy changes that can improve the cosmic landscape for individuals living with arthritis.

Cosmic Technology: Embrace the cosmic wonders of technology! Explore cosmic apps, websites, or social media platforms that provide cosmic resources, cosmic tracking tools, and cosmic inspiration for managing arthritis. From cosmic exercise apps to cosmic meditation guides, technology can be a cosmic companion in your arthritis journey.

Cosmic Hobbies and Interests: Engage in cosmic hobbies or activities that bring you joy and help you connect with like-minded cosmic individuals. Whether it's joining a cosmic book club, attending cosmic art classes, or participating in cosmic sports teams, these cosmic endeavors can create new cosmic friendships and provide a cosmic sense of belonging.

Cosmic Service Animals: Consider the cosmic companionship of a service animal. Trained cosmic service dogs or other animals can provide cosmic assistance and emotional support, helping to alleviate cosmic stress and providing a cosmic sense of comfort.

Cosmic Laughter: Remember, laughter is cosmic medicine! Surround yourself with cosmic people who bring joy and humor into your cosmic world. Share cosmic jokes, indulge in cosmic comedy shows, and find cosmic reasons to laugh. Laughter can lighten the cosmic load and strengthen the cosmic bonds of your support system.

In the cosmic battle against arthritis, building a support system is like assembling your cosmic team of superheroes. Each member plays a vital role in your cosmic journey, providing support, guidance, and cosmic companionship. So, embrace the cosmic connections and let your support system be your cosmic allies as you navigate the cosmic cosmos of arthritis.

# Embracing strengths and talents

When it comes to arthritis, it's easy to focus on the challenges and limitations it brings. However, it's equally important to embrace your strengths and talents as cosmic superpowers that can help you navigate the cosmic terrain of arthritis. So, let's embark on a cosmic journey of self-discovery and celebrate the cosmic abilities that make you unique.

Cosmic Adaptability: Arthritis may present cosmic challenges, but it also sparks your cosmic adaptability. You develop cosmic problem-solving skills and find creative ways to accomplish cosmic tasks. Embrace your ability to adapt and conquer the cosmic obstacles that come your way.

Cosmic Resilience: Living with arthritis requires cosmic resilience. Each cosmic flare-up or setback provides an opportunity to bounce back stronger. Embrace your inner superhero and let your cosmic resilience shine through in the face of cosmic adversity.

Cosmic Empathy: Arthritis grants you cosmic empathy, as you understand the cosmic struggles faced by others living with chronic conditions. Your empathetic nature can create cosmic connections and allow you to provide cosmic support to those in need.

Cosmic Patience: Arthritis teaches you cosmic patience. You become a master of pacing yourself, recognizing your limits, and practicing self-care. Embrace your cosmic patience and let it guide you on your cosmic journey to manage arthritis.

Cosmic Creativity: Living with arthritis fosters cosmic creativity. From finding alternative ways to perform daily tasks to adapting your hobbies to accommodate your needs, your cosmic creativity shines through. Embrace your cosmic creativity and let it bring joy and fulfillment to your life.

Cosmic Persistence: Dealing with arthritis requires cosmic persistence. Despite the challenges, you keep pushing forward, seeking solutions, and advocating for your needs. Your cosmic persistence is a testament to your determination and strength.

Cosmic Mindfulness: Arthritis encourages cosmic mindfulness, as you learn to listen to your body, recognize its signals, and respond accordingly. Embrace the cosmic practice of mindfulness and let it bring cosmic peace and awareness to your life.

Cosmic Adaptations: You discover cosmic adaptations that enhance your daily life. Whether it's using assistive devices, implementing ergonomic workstations, or incorporating joint-friendly exercises, you find ways to optimize your cosmic abilities and maintain independence.

Cosmic Advocacy: Embrace your cosmic advocacy skills as you raise awareness about arthritis and advocate for improved cosmic access to healthcare, resources, and support. Your voice has the cosmic power to make a difference in the lives of others living with arthritis.

Cosmic Humor: Laughter is cosmic medicine, and your ability to find humor in challenging situations is a cosmic superpower. Embrace your cosmic sense of humor and let it lighten the cosmic load, bringing joy and positivity into your life and the lives of others.

Remember, embracing your strengths and talents is not about denying the challenges of arthritis but acknowledging your cosmic abilities to overcome them. Each cosmic strength you possess is a valuable asset in managing arthritis and living a fulfilling life. So, celebrate your cosmic powers, embrace your uniqueness, and let them guide you on your cosmic journey with arthritis.

# Conclusion

In conclusion, arthritis is a cosmic journey that presents its fair share of challenges. However, by understanding arthritis and exploring its various aspects, we can navigate this cosmic terrain with grace, resilience, and even a little humor.

Throughout this cosmic adventure, we have delved into the cosmic depths of arthritis, gaining a greater understanding of its causes, symptoms, and impact on daily life. We have explored the cosmic strategies for managing pain, improving mobility, and nurturing our mental well-being. We have discovered the cosmic importance of a healthy lifestyle, including exercise, diet, and sleep. And we have recognized the cosmic significance of building a support system, embracing our strengths, and seeking proper treatment.

Living with arthritis is no cosmic joke, but injecting a little humor into the journey can lighten the cosmic load. It allows us to find moments of levity amidst the challenges, to laugh at ourselves when we stumble, and to maintain a positive outlook despite the cosmic obstacles we face.

Remember, you are a cosmic superhero on this arthritis journey. Embrace your cosmic adaptability, resilience, and patience. Harness your cosmic creativity, empathy, and advocacy skills. Celebrate your cosmic strengths and talents, for they are the cosmic superpowers that will guide you forward.

As we conclude our exploration of understanding arthritis, let's embark on this cosmic adventure with a newfound sense of empowerment. Let's face each cosmic challenge head-on, armed with knowledge, strategies, and a dash of humor. Together, we can create a cosmic community that supports and uplifts one another in the face of arthritis.

Arthritis may be a cosmic companion, but it doesn't define who we are. We are more than our cosmic condition. We are cosmic beings with cosmic dreams, aspirations, and limitless potential. Arthritis may change the cosmic landscape, but it cannot extinguish the cosmic spark within us.

So, let's embrace this cosmic journey with open arms, knowing that we have the cosmic strength to persevere, the cosmic wisdom to adapt, and the cosmic support of those around us. We can live fulfilling, cosmic lives despite arthritis's cosmic challenges.

Remember, as we travel through this cosmic universe of arthritis, we are never alone. There are cosmic healthcare professionals, support groups, and communities ready to lend a helping hand and cosmic support.

Arthritis may be a cosmic adventure we didn't ask for, but with the right knowledge, tools, and mindset, we can navigate its cosmic terrain and thrive. Let's celebrate the cosmic abilities within us, find joy in the cosmic moments, and continue to grow, learn, and inspire others along the way.

Arthritis is just one cosmic chapter in our cosmic story. Let's make it a chapter filled with resilience, laughter, and cosmic triumphs. Together, we can create a cosmic legacy that defies the limitations of arthritis and celebrates the indomitable cosmic spirit within us all.

# Recap of key takeaways

As we reach the end of our cosmic journey exploring the vast realm of arthritis, let's take a moment to recap the key takeaways from our exploration. After all, a cosmic adventure like this deserves a cosmic summary!

First and foremost, understanding arthritis is crucial. We've learned that arthritis is not just one cosmic entity but encompasses various types, such as osteoarthritis, rheumatoid arthritis, and psoriatic arthritis. Each type has its cosmic characteristics and affects the cosmic body in different ways.

Arthritis can have a cosmic impact on daily life, affecting mobility, sleep, mental health, and work. But fear not, for there are cosmic strategies to manage arthritis symptoms and mitigate their cosmic impact. From physical therapy and exercise to dietary changes and stress reduction techniques, we have explored a cosmic array of approaches to help us navigate this cosmic challenge.

Building a support system is cosmic armor in the face of arthritis. Whether it's seeking support from healthcare professionals, joining support groups, or connecting with loved ones, having cosmic allies by our side can make the journey much more manageable. We've also discovered the importance of embracing our cosmic strengths and talents, finding humor in the cosmic absurdities, and advocating for ourselves in the cosmic realm of arthritis.

Treatment and proper healthcare play a cosmic role in managing arthritis. Medications, both prescription and over-the-counter, can alleviate pain and reduce inflammation. However, it's important to consider potential side effects and cosmic risks associated with these treatments. We've also explored natural remedies and alternative therapies, recognizing that there is a cosmic spectrum of options available to complement conventional treatments.

Maintaining a healthy lifestyle is cosmic medicine for arthritis. Regular exercise, such as low-impact activities and strength training, can improve mobility and reduce pain. A cosmic diet rich in anti-inflammatory foods, while avoiding cosmic culprits like processed foods and excessive sugar, can also play a significant cosmic role in managing arthritis symptoms.

Sleep, oh cosmic sleep! It is a cosmic necessity for our well-being. We've learned that arthritis can disrupt our cosmic slumber, but implementing strategies such as creating a cosmic sleep routine and using aids like pillows and mattress toppers can help improve our cosmic rest.

Arthritis is not just a physical condition; it impacts our mental health as well. Cosmic strategies like stress reduction techniques, mindfulness, and seeking professional support can help us navigate the cosmic emotional challenges that arthritis presents.

And finally, let's not forget the cosmic power of humor. Laughter is cosmic medicine that can lighten the cosmic load and bring cosmic joy amidst the challenges of arthritis. So, let's embrace the cosmic absurdities, find humor in the cosmic moments, and keep a positive cosmic outlook.

In conclusion, understanding arthritis is a cosmic journey that requires knowledge, resilience, and a dash of humor. By implementing cosmic strategies, building a cosmic support system, and seeking proper treatment, we can navigate the cosmic landscape of arthritis with grace and cosmic triumph. Remember, you are a cosmic superhero on this cosmic adventure, equipped with the wisdom and tools to overcome the challenges of arthritis and embrace a fulfilling cosmic life. So, let's embark on this cosmic journey together, armed with knowledge, resilience, and a cosmic sense of humor.

# Encouragement to seek treatment and support for arthritis

Imagine this cosmic scenario: You're the captain of your own spaceship, exploring the vast universe of life. Suddenly, you encounter a celestial body called arthritis. It's not the most welcoming cosmic neighbor, but fear not! With the right cosmic guidance, you can navigate this cosmic challenge and conquer it like the cosmic hero you are.

Arthritis is a cosmic condition that affects millions of people across the galaxy. It can cause cosmic discomfort, pain, and limitations in your cosmic activities. But here's the cosmic truth: seeking treatment and support is the cosmic key to managing arthritis and living a fulfilling cosmic life.

First and foremost, don't be afraid to consult cosmic healthcare professionals. They are the cosmic experts who can guide you through the cosmic maze of arthritis. Whether it's a rheumatologist, physical therapist, or occupational therapist, they have the cosmic knowledge and experience to help you find cosmic relief. So, don't hesitate to schedule your cosmic appointments and let these cosmic experts guide you on your journey.

In addition to professional guidance, building a cosmic support system is essential. Surround yourself with cosmic allies who understand and empathize with your cosmic battles. Join support groups, both online and in-person, where you can connect with other cosmic warriors facing similar challenges. Share your cosmic triumphs and struggles, and find cosmic solace in the cosmic camaraderie.

Now, let's talk about treatments. Medications can be cosmic allies in managing arthritis symptoms. From nonsteroidal anti-inflammatory drugs (NSAIDs) to disease-modifying antirheumatic drugs (DMARDs), there's a cosmic arsenal of medications available to help you tame the cosmic inflammation and pain. But remember, cosmic hero, consult your healthcare professional for the right cosmic prescription.

But wait, there's more! Cosmic lifestyle modifications can also make a cosmic difference. Regular exercise, cosmic warriors, can improve joint flexibility and cosmic strength. It's time to engage in cosmic activities that bring you joy. Cosmic walking, swimming, or yoga can be great choices. Just make sure to listen to your cosmic body and find activities that are both enjoyable and cosmic-friendly.

In the cosmic realm of diet, small cosmic changes can have a big impact. Incorporating anti-inflammatory foods like cosmic fruits, vegetables, and omega-3 fatty acids can support your cosmic battle against arthritis. And don't forget to stay cosmic-hydrated! Hydration is cosmic fuel for your joints.

Last but not least, let's sprinkle a little cosmic humor on this cosmic journey. Laughter is cosmic medicine that can lift your spirits and bring cosmic joy. Embrace the cosmic absurdities, find humor in the cosmic moments, and let laughter be your cosmic ally in overcoming the challenges of arthritis.

So, my cosmic friend, don't let arthritis hold you back. Seek treatment, build your cosmic support system, and make cosmic lifestyle changes that support your journey. Remember, you're a cosmic hero with the power to conquer any cosmic challenge that comes your way.

In conclusion, seeking treatment and support for arthritis is not a sign of cosmic weakness but a cosmic act of empowerment. You deserve to live a cosmic life free from the cosmic burdens of arthritis. So, let's embark on this cosmic journey together, armed with cosmic knowledge, cosmic support, and a cosmic sense of humor. The universe awaits, and your cosmic triumph over arthritis is within reach.

# Have Questions / Comments?

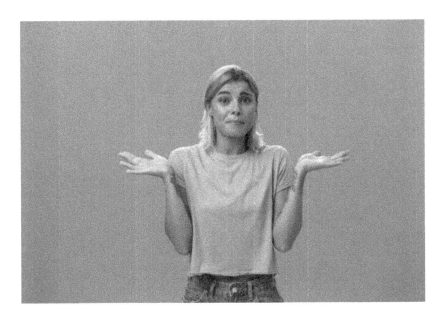

1

This book was designed to cover as much as possible but I know I have probably missed something, or some new amazing discovery that has just come out.

If you notice something missing or have a question that I failed to answer, please get in touch and let me know. If I can, I will email you an answer and also update the book so others can also benefit from it.

Thanks For Being Awesome :)

Submit Your Questions / Comments At:

## https://go.xspurts.com/questions

# Get Another Book Free

We love writing and have produced a huge number of books.

For being one of our amazing readers, we would love to offer you another book we have created, 100% free.

To claim this limited time special offer, simply go to the site below and enter your name and email address.

You will then receive one of my great books, direct to your email account, 100% free!

**https://go.xspurts.com/free-book-offer**

---

# Also by Kian M. Hart

Printed in July 2023
by Rotomail Italia S.p.A., Vignate (MI) - Italy